First Edition

Pharmacology of Recreational Drugs

The Neurology of How Drugs Work

by Donald Slish

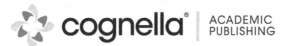

Bassim Hamadeh, CEO and Publisher
Kassie Graves, Director of Acquisitions and Sales
Jamie Giganti, Senior Managing Editor
Miguel Macias, Senior Graphic Designer
John Remington, Acquisitions Editor
Monika Dziamka, Project Editor
Brian Fahey, Licensing Associate
Berenice Quirino, Associate Production Editor
Joyce Lue, Interior Designer

ISBN: 978-1-5165-0441-1 (pbk) / 978-1-5165-0442-8 (br)

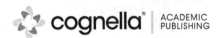

Contents

Chapter 2: Pharmacodynamics I   19

Chapter 3: Pharmacodynamics II   31

Chapter 6: Cognition   73

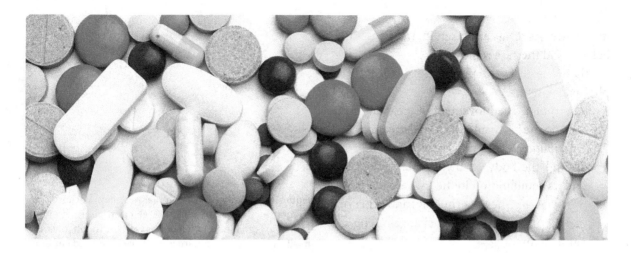

Chapter 1:
Pharmacokinetics

Pharmacology

Pharmacology, broadly defined, is the study of how drugs work. The root *pharm* comes from the Greek word *pharmakon*, which means both drug and poison. The Swiss-German Renaissance physician Paracelsus said, "Poison is in everything, and no thing is without poison. The dosage makes it either a poison or a remedy." Stated another way, the difference between a drug and a poison is the dose. For example, water is vital to life. Under average conditions, a person can only live three to five days without water. However, drinking six liters of water in an hour will kill a person. This dose of water dilutes the blood and causes swelling of the brain, resulting in loss of consciousness, cessation of breathing, and death.

Part of the discipline of pharmacology concerns studying the biochemical and physiological mechanisms of action of drugs. This is called *pharmacodynamics*. Most of this book is dedicated to pharmacodynamics. However,

another important aspect of how drugs work is pharmacokinetics, which also greatly affects the action of drugs as well as the addiction potential of some drugs. That is the topic of this first chapter.

Pharmacokinetics

Pharmacokinetics is the study of how drugs get into the bloodstream, how they are distributed, and how they are eliminated. These basic principles apply to all drugs but vary based on the properties of the drug in question.

Kinetics is the study of the rate of change (e.g., change in concentration per unit time). Whether the drug is increasing in the body (absorption) or decreasing (metabolism and elimination), it is always changing. The change of a drug's concentration in the body over time affects the time to the onset of effects, the duration of action of the drug, and the persistence of the drug in body (for detection). Any drug taken into the body will eventually be removed, despite stories of drugs (e.g., LSD) being stored long-term in the body. This is part of the body's effort to maintain homeostasis, or a steady state—a body maintaining its balance. As drugs are taken in, they upset the balance and they are removed.

There are four processes involved in pharmacokinetics:

1. *Absorption.* The movement of the drug from outside the body into the bloodstream.
2. *Distribution.* The movement of the drug around the body by the circulatory system and its equilibration in the tissues.
3. *Metabolism.* The liver (mainly) and other organs acting on the drug to change its chemical structure.
4. *Elimination.* Movement of the drug and its metabolites out of the body, usually by the kidneys into the urine.

Absorption and distribution determine the rate of the onset of effects of the drug. Metabolism and elimination determine the duration of its action and how long the drug can be detected in the urine or blood after it has been taken.

Absorption

The rate of absorption depends on two things: the route of administration and the polarity of the drug. The polarity is based on the structure of the drug itself, and the route of administration is determined by the user. Both have impacts on all aspects of pharmacokinetics.

Polarity

The *polarity* of the drug determines whether the drug is soluble in water or lipid. Water is a very polar molecule because it has strong partial charges associated with it (see Figure 1.1). Lipids are mainly composed of carbon-hydrogen bonds, which lack polarity. As such, they are called *nonpolar*.

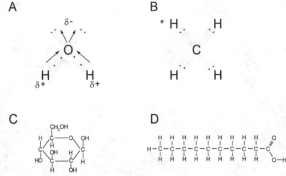

Figure 1.1 A. Water is a very polar molecule because the oxygen at the center pulls the electron clouds (represented in light blue) of their bonds with hydrogen towards itself. This produces a partial negative charge (d⁻) at one end and a partial positive charge (d⁺) at the other. B. In a nonpolar molecule like methane (shown here), the central carbon atom is symmetrically surrounded by identical atoms (hydrogen). As such, there are no poles. C. Molecules like glucose shown here have many polar functional groups (OH), which make them polar. D. Fatty acids are mainly composed of carbon-hydrogen bonds and are therefore non-polar.

One way to measure polarity is with the lipid partition coefficient (see Figure 1.2). Drugs are organic molecules (i.e., carbon-based), and their structures vary greatly. They can have functional groups, like amines, alcohols, or acids that add full or partial charges to the molecule. Charges make the molecule more polar and therefore more soluble in water. In a mixture that contains both water and oil, drugs with a strongly polar functional groups will preferentially dissolve (or partition) into the water layer, although some will also be in the oil (see Figure 1.2A). Drugs without strongly polar functional groups will preferentially partition into the oil layer.

This has an important effect on the absorption of a drug, because the plasma membranes of cells are made of phospholipids, which are very nonpolar. Drugs that are soluble in lipid pass through this easily (see Figure 1.2B). In routes of administration that involve dissolving through membranes (e.g., snorting a drug),

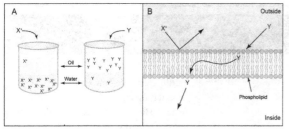

Figure 1.2 A. To determine how polar or nonpolar a molecule is, it is equilibrated in a solution that is half water and half oil. The amount of the molecule in each portion is then measured and compared. Here X+ represents a polar molecule and Y represents a non-polar molecule. B. The lipid bilayer of cell membranes blocks the entry of polar molecules (X+) but allow nonpolar molecules (Y) to enter.

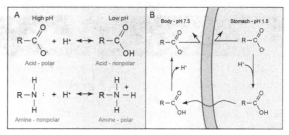

Figure 1.3 A. Many organic molecules have either acid groups (COOH) or amine groups (NH2). These can change in charge depending on the pH of the solution. B. The diffusion of a molecule across a membrane can be affected by the different pH in each compartment. Here an acid becomes protonated and uncharged in the low pH of the stomach. This allows it to diffuse into the body and become unprotonated by the relatively higher pH there, trapping it in the body.

nonpolar drugs diffuse into the body easily. Drugs that are polar have difficulty passing through cell membranes and do not enter well this way. They need to be administered in a different way (e.g., by injection). Polarity will also affect the ability of a drug to enter the brain from the bloodstream, as is discussed below in the section on distribution.

A factor that complicates this is the fact that acid and amine functional groups can change in polarity, depending on the pH of the solution that they are in (see Figure 1.3A). The *pH* of a solution is its H^+ concentration. In low pH (high H^+ concentration), amines pick up a H^+ and become positively charged, while acids pick up a H^+ and become neutral (nonpolar). In high pH (low H^+ concentration), the opposite happens; amines become neutral, and acids become charged. This is important in the oral administration of drugs where the pH between the stomach and blood and between the small intestine and blood is very different (see Figure 1.3B). It is also important in the use of "free-base" drugs such as crack cocaine, as it affects the absorption of the drug.

Route of Administration

The *route of administration* is the method by which the drug enters the body. This can greatly affect the rate at which the drug peaks in the bloodstream, how long it takes to reach the peak, the drug's concentration at peak, and how long the drug lasts in the system. There are five ways in which a drug is usually administered: orally, rectally, parenterally (by injection), by inhalation, and by diffusion across membranes. Each has its advantages and disadvantages (see Table 1.1).

Oral Administration

Oral administration (*per os*, or PO in medical terminology) is when a drug is taken by mouth. This is the slowest means of absorption but the easiest route of administration. Drugs taken orally can take minutes to hours to enter the bloodstream. This slow absorption is often preferred medically, because adverse effects can be recognized and countered before it is too late. However, in an emergency situation, oral administration may be too slow.

Table 1.1 Advantages and Disadvantages of Different Routes of Administration

	Advantages	Disadvantages
Oral	Slowest Easy Longest lasting Extended release	Slowest Acidic, destroy some drugs Stomach upset Variable: food, first pass, bioavailability Multiple dosing risk
Rectal	Slow Easy Little first-pass	Slow Stigmatized
Parenteral	Very fast Closely controlled dosing Avoid absorption barriers	Very fast Infection Collapsed veins
Inhalation	Fastest Closely controlled dosing	Fastest (addiction potential) Burning (PAHs)
Topical	Easy Avoids first pass Extended release	Local tissue damage Only nonpolar drugs

The stomach can provide challenges for oral administration. The stomach is very acidic, with a very low pH (between 1.5 and 3.5). This can cause rapid absorption of acidic drugs such as aspirin, which become nonpolar (see Figure 1.3B). This causes a very high concentration of the drug in the stomach lining and can lead to stomach upset, which is a side effect common to many drugs. Also, the low pH can destroy some drugs; a drug given orally must be stable in low pH. Protein drugs (e.g., insulin) cannot be given orally, as they will be digested by the enzymes and the low pH in the stomach.

The amount of food in the stomach has an important effect on the rate of absorption. Most of a drug will be absorbed in the small intestine, so the amount of time a drug stays in the stomach adds to the time it takes to be absorbed. A mostly empty stomach will move what little it contains into the small intestine quickly. A full stomach will churn and mix its contents, slowly releasing small amounts as the small intestine is ready for more. For this reason, a drug taken on an empty stomach will be passed on to the small intestine and absorbed faster than a drug taken on a full stomach would. This increases the variability in absorption rate of an orally consumed drug.

As stated above, most of the absorption occurs in the small intestine. The small intestine has many blood vessels and is specially designed for absorption. A unique aspect of its vasculature is that all of the blood that leaves the small intestine goes directly to the liver, instead of back to the heart, as in all other organs (see Figure 1.4). This is called the *hepatic portal circulation*. It ensures that anything absorbed in the intestines goes though the liver before it enters the main circulation. The role of the liver, as will be discussed later, is to detoxify the blood.

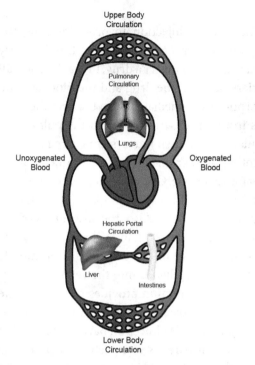

Figure 1.4 The circulatory system has two main circuits. The pulmonary circuit takes unoxygenated blood (in blue) from the right side of the heart to the lungs to be oxygenated and back to the heart. The oxygenated blood (in red) is then pumped by the left side of the heart into the systemic circuit, which includes the upper body circulation (including the brain) and the lower body circulation. Note that blood of the systemic circuit that enters the intestines goes to the liver before returning to the heart (hepatic portal circulation).

The hepatic portal circulation is an evolutionary adaptation that filters out many toxins commonly found in food. This process leads to a phenomenon called the *first-pass effect*. Any drugs taken orally are acted on by the liver before they enter the bloodstream. Not all drugs are broken down here, but some are changed quite a bit, making them either less or more effective. This complicates oral administration in that it adds a level of unpredictability to dosing. In addition, different people have different levels of liver metabolism (as will be discussed below), so the dose given is not necessarily the dose received. Also, it limits oral administration to drugs that

are not extensively metabolized by the liver. If most of a drug is metabolized in the first pass, a different means of administration may be used.

The bioavailability of a drug adds further unpredictability to the dosing of drugs. *Bioavailability* refers to the amount of the drug that is absorbed in the intestines. Some drugs—for example, curare—are not absorbed at all from the intestines and pass out of the digestive system. The bioavailability of some drugs may differ between people, adding more variability.

Bioavailability can be used as an advantage in the compounding of drugs. If a drug is needed for long periods at a relatively constant dose, it can be compounded into a controlled-release formulation. This compound is a drug bound up with other chemicals that block the drug's absorption (usually physically). The compounding chemicals break down slowly as the mixture passes through the small intestine, releasing the drug over time. In this way, a drug that would normally last at an effective dose for four hours can be made into an extended-release formulation (ER) to last twelve or twenty-four hours.

One of the dangers of oral administration for recreational drugs is that users can underestimate the time that it takes for the drug to peak. This can lead to dangerous multiple dosing. When users do not feel effects in thirty minutes or more, they may take another dose, assuming that the first dose was too low. By the time the second dose peaks, the user may require medical attention. This is common for drugs that peak slowly, such as ecstasy, LSD, and edible cannabis.

Rectal Administration

The rectum is the short end portion of the intestinal tract that stores feces for disposal. Rectal insertion is another means of administering a drug.

Pharmaceutically, this is often done by compounding a drug into a rectal suppository. However, any drug can be inserted and absorbed in the rectum, and this is done clinically by dissolving the drug and administering via a rectal catheter.

There are several advantages to rectal absorption. It can be useful if the patient is vomiting, unconscious, or unable to swallow. Also, it is useful in pediatrics because it can be difficult to administer oral drugs to children due to non-compliance. Rectal suppositories produce a slow means of absorption, although it is usually faster than oral administration. Rectal absorption avoids the first-pass effect because only one-third of veins leaving the rectum flow into the hepatic portal circulation.

Parenteral Administration

Parenteral administration means injection of a dissolved drug directly into the body via a hypodermic needle (see Figure 1.5). There are three common types of parenteral administration: intravenous (IV), intramuscular (IM), and subcutaneous (SC). Each has slightly different advantages and times to peak absorption.

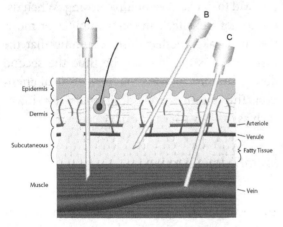

Figure 1.5 A. Intramuscular injection (IM). B. Subcutaneous injection (SC). C. Intravenous injection (IV).

Intravenous injection involves injecting the drug directly into a surface vein. This is a very rapid way to administer a drug, in that it avoids all barriers between the drug and the bloodstream; absorption is immediate. From the vein the drug goes to the heart, from there to the pulmonary circulation, and then into systemic circulation.

Intramuscular injection involves injecting the drug into a muscle. One advantage of this method over IV is that it is easier to inject into a muscle than it is into a vein. Also, the absorption of the drug is slightly slower than IV, because the drug must first diffuse into capillaries in the muscle and from the capillaries into the veins. Similarly, subcutaneous injection provides an easier route than IV and a slower absorption. Another advantage that SC and IM injection have over IV is that there are still barriers to infection to overcome in the skin and muscle. Contaminated needles inject infectious agents directly into the circulation when drugs are injected via an IV.

One major advantage of injection is that it avoids absorption barriers. This means that the drug peaks very quickly. This is an advantage in emergency situations or any time the onset of effects needs to be closely controlled (e.g., during surgery), as injections avoid the bioavailability and first-pass problems of oral administration. Finally, if the environment of the stomach is hostile to the drug (e.g., as with insulin), injection is a more effective way to administer the drug.

One of the disadvantages of injection is the possibility of infection. Even under optimal conditions, bacteria and viruses can be carried under the skin and avoid the defenses there. This is especially a problem with street drugs. IV drug users often pass viruses such as HIV and hepatitis when they share needles. Also, impurities in street drugs can cause irritation and break down tissues.

Another disadvantage is that the drug level peaks almost instantly, and the effects come on very quickly. If the recipient has an allergic or other adverse reaction to the drug, it may occur too rapidly to prevent it. This rapid onset of the drug's effect also increases the "rush" of drugs such as heroin and cocaine, which increases their addiction potential.

Finally, repeated injection in veins eventually collapses the vessel. Every injection causes damage that results in scar formation. Infrequent injection poses no danger, but scar tissue and clots build up from repeated injection in the same spot. This damage eventually closes the vessel, and without blood flowing through it, the vessel collapses. IV drug abusers move from one vein to another as routes for administration become harder and harder to find. Eventually they graduate to injecting in the feet, ankles, groin, neck, and sometimes the soft tissue around the eye.

Inhalation

Inhalation is a method that is used for drugs that are volatile (inhalation anesthetics, organic solvents, etc.) or can be volatilized by heating (cannabis, methamphetamine, crack cocaine, etc.). This is the fastest means of drug absorption.

The respiratory system is composed of the trachea (windpipe), bronchi, bronchioles, and alveoli (see Figure 1.6). The trachea, bronchi, and bronchioles make up the pathway that inhaled air follows; little absorption occurs here. The alveoli are blind sacs at the end of the bronchioles. These are highly vascularized, and the exchange of gases between the inhaled air and the blood in the capillaries occurs here. This exchange is passive and based on the concentration gradient of the gases involved. Carbon dioxide (CO_2) is higher in concentration in the blood, so it diffuses out of the blood and into the alveolus. Oxygen (O_2) is higher in concentration in the inspired air, so it diffuses into

the blood in the capillaries, where it is bound by the hemoglobin in the red blood cells.

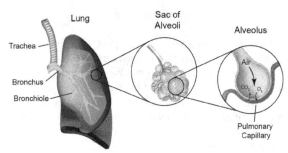

Figure 1.6 Air enters the lungs through the trachea and divides to the left and right lungs via bronchi. Each bronchus divides further to for bronchioles that end in a sac of alveoli. Alveoli and highly vascularized and gas exchange occurs between the thin cells of the alveolus and the capillary.

In the same way, inhaled drugs can diffuse between the inspired air in the alveolus and the blood in the capillaries, depending on their concentration. For example, nitrous oxide (N_2O) is safely administered clinically by controlling its concentration in the inspired air (see Figure 1.7). The N_2O diffuses into the bloodstream until the concentration is the same on either side of the alveolus membrane. The concentration in the blood is then the same as the concentration in the inspired air. When the N_2O is removed from the inspired air, it diffuses back out of the blood, into the alveolus, and is exhaled.

Drugs that are volatile at body temperature, such as ethyl alcohol, will diffuse out of the body via the alveoli. Thus, the breathalyzer can approximate the concentration of ethanol in the blood by measuring its concentration in expired air. Drugs that are not normally volatile at body temperature (e.g., cocaine and methamphetamine) will be absorbed rapidly in the alveoli when heated and inhaled, but little will diffuse out via this mechanism.

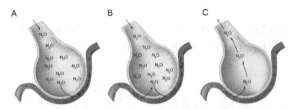

Figure 1.7 The absorption of a drug in the alveoli is based on its concentration gradient. A. When the inspired air has a higher concentration than the blood, the gas (nitrous oxide, N2O) diffuses into the blood. B. With time, the concentration of drug in the blood will equilibrate with its concentration in the inspired air and there is no net movement. C. When the drug is removed from the inspired air, the net movement is out of the blood and the drug is exhaled.

Inhalation is the fastest means of absorption, because drugs absorbed through the lungs go to the heart via the pulmonary circuit and are then pumped directly into the systemic circuit. Inhaled drugs such as crack cocaine can peak in the brain in five to seven seconds; this is about half the time it takes for injected drugs to reach the brain.

The ability of a drug to rapidly reach the brain can be an advantage clinically when drugs need to be administered quickly. Also, the rapid equilibrium between inhaled gases and the blood allows doctors to carefully control the dose in the brain. In terms of recreational drugs, this method is preferable to IV administration, with faster results. However, the rapid onset of a drug's effect can initiate precipitous allergic or overdose reactions and is associated with a greater addiction potential of drugs (this will be discussed in Chapter 9, CNS Stimulants).

Another negative aspect to inhalation occurs when the volatilization is achieved by burning, as with tobacco or cannabis. The burning of the plant material provides the heat that volatilizes the drug. However, this incomplete burning produces polyaromatic hydrocarbons (PAHs), which are carcinogenic. Volatilization methods that do not include burning, such as vaping, are safer.

Topical Administration

In topical administration, the drug is absorbed directly across a layer of cells exposed to the environment. This includes transdermal, intranasal, transvaginal, and oral absorption. Oral absorption here means absorption through the membranes in the mouth rather than after swallowing. Some examples of topical administration are snorting cocaine, sublingual use of nitroglycerine (for angina), sucking opioid lollipops (for children), and applying transdermal patches (e.g., nicotine or birth control).

Advantages of this route are ease of administration and rapid absorption. It also avoids the first-pass effect seen with oral administration. The duration of action of the drug can be very short, as with other rapid means of absorption, because it is controlled by the metabolism and elimination of the drug and not its absorption (this is described further below). An exception to this is the transdermal patch. Transdermal patches are designed to release the drug to the skin surface slowly (see Figure 1.8). This form of controlled release or extended release can deliver the drug at a constant rate for hours to weeks.

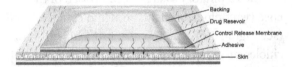

Figure 1.8 The transdermal patch is composed of several layers. The adhesive and backing layers hold the patch together and adhere it to the skin. The drug reservoir contains and releases the drug. The control release membrane hampers the diffusion of the drug from the reservoir to attend a constant release of the drug and absorption by the body.

One disadvantage of this method is that the drug can cause local damage at the site of the absorption. This area experiences the highest concentration of the drug, so tissues here can be damaged. This is common in the nasal administration of cocaine. Another disadvantage of this route is that only relatively nonpolar drugs can be absorbed this way. Drugs absorbed topically must first diffuse into and then through the cells at the surface. The lipid membrane of cells creates a significant barrier to polar molecules. Only nonpolar drugs can do this at an appreciable rate.

Distribution

Once the drug has been absorbed into the capillaries, it is distributed by the cardiovascular system. There are two circuits to the cardiovascular system, the pulmonary circuit and the systemic circuit (see Figure 1.4). The pulmonary circuit takes blood from the heart to the lungs for the exchange of O_2 and CO_2. The systemic circuit takes this oxygenated blood to the rest of the body.

The Cardiovascular System

Arteries are the blood vessels that take the blood away from the heart. As the blood gets further from the heart, the arteries branch into smaller and smaller vessels, first into arterioles and then to the tiny, delicate capillaries. The walls of capillaries are only one endothelial cell thick and are arranged in a network throughout the tissues. The exchange of gases and other materials occurs in this network of tiny vessels (the capillary bed), both in the tissues of the body and in the alveoli of the lung. Capillaries join to form venules (i.e., small veins). These venules join to form veins, and the veins join to form the major veins of the body that empty into the heart.

In most tissues of the body, the endothelial cells in capillary beds have small gaps between them

that allow water and dissolved molecules (such as ions, glucose, and polar drugs) to escape the capillaries and enter the tissues (see Figure 1.9A). For this reason, once a drug has been absorbed and reached equilibrium in the blood, it is distributed equally to the extracellular fluid of all cells of the body, and they all experience the same concentration of the drug. This is also true of maternal-fetal circulation. Drugs and toxins in the maternal blood will equilibrate with the fetal blood, and the fetus will be exposed to any drugs taken by the mother. This has the potential for acute toxicity in the fetus (often due to vasoconstriction and lack of O_2) and teratogenic effects (birth defects).

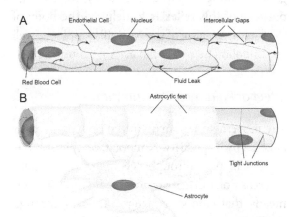

Figure 1.9 A. There are small gaps between the endothelial cells of most capillaries of the body. This allows polar dissolved molecules and ions to leave the capillaries and equilibrate with the extracellular fluid surrounding the cells. B. The endothelial cells of the brain are joined by tight junctions that don't allow fluid to escape. In addition, astrocytes extend processes that wrap around the capillaries, which form a nonpolar barrier between the blood stream and the capillaries.

One important exception to this distribution is in the brain. Here the gaps between the endothelial cells are sealed by tight junctions that do not allow polar substances to pass. In addition, helper cells called *astrocytes* (described in Chapter 2) send processes out to surround the capillaries and seal them off (see Figure 1.9B). These processes are basically the plasma membrane of the astrocyte wrapping multiple times around the vessels to produce a nonpolar barrier between the vessel and the brain tissue. This is called the *blood-brain barrier* (*BBB*), and its purpose is to protect the brain from toxins. However, nonpolar molecules, being able to dissolve into and through membranes, can pass through this barrier. This affects the distribution of polar and nonpolar drugs.

One area of the brain with a reduced BBB is the area postrema in the medulla (in the brain stem), also called the *chemical trigger zone* (*CTZ*). This is the area in the medulla that triggers vomiting when activated by toxins. The purpose of this reflex is to help rid the body of the toxins. Because of the weak BBB, polar as well as nonpolar chemicals can activate vomiting.

Effect of Polarity on Distribution

The movement of a drug in the body is strongly affected by its polarity. Nonpolar, or lipid soluble, drugs can pass through cell membranes easily, whereas polar drugs cannot (see Figure 1.2). This means that nonpolar drugs can pass through the BBB and enter the brain. Indeed, for a recreational drug to have any effect, it must be at least somewhat nonpolar or else it will be excluded from the brain.

Another phenomenon seen with nonpolar drugs is partitioning into the fatty tissues of the body. The drug's preference to dissolve in lipid causes it to avoid the water solution of the blood and accumulate in fatty tissues, which reduces its plasma concentration. This is explained by the two-compartment model (see Figure 1.10). The lipid compartment represents cell membranes and adipose tissue; the aqueous compartment represents the blood and cytoplasm of cells. As the drug is eliminated from the blood by the liver

and kidneys, its concentration there drops and it leaches out of the fatty tissues into the plasma. This increases the time the drug is in the body and allows for detection of the drug in the plasma and urine long after the effects of the drug have dissipated.

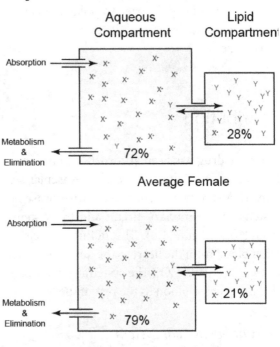

Figure 1.10 The body can be imagined to be composed of two compartments. The aqueous compartment represents the blood, extracellular fluid and intracellular fluid of cells. The lipid compartment represents adipose tissue (fat cells) and the phospholipid membranes of cells. The relative proportion of these two compartments varies by gender. A polar drug (X+) preferentially partitions into the aqueous compartment and is easily removed by the kidneys. A nonpolar drug (Y) preferentially partitions into the lipid compartment, decreasing its concentration in the blood. As it is removed from the aqueous compartment, the nonpolar drug slowly leaches out of the lipid compartment and is eliminated.

The duration of the drug's action can also be affected by this partitioning. If a very nonpolar drug is taken by inhalation, on its first pass of distribution it will partition into the brain (which is very fatty). The effect of the drug is then much higher than would have been predicted by the dose taken because it is concentrated where it has its desired effect. However, over a short period of time, the drug leaches out of the brain and the effect goes away. This is particularly true of inhalation anesthetics and crack cocaine.

Metabolism

Metabolism, or *biotransformation*, is done by enzymes and can occur in the stomach, plasma, intestine, kidneys, or brain. However, most metabolism occurs in the liver, which is the main organ for detoxification of the blood. Enzymes in the liver chemically modify lipid-soluble drugs to make them polar. This metabolism is an attempt to make the drugs more water soluble so that the kidneys can eliminate them. It also helps exclude them from the brain because of the BBB.

An important thing to remember about this process is that it is not specific to any particular drug; it generally cleanses the blood of toxins. Many drugs are inactivated by these enzymes; however, some can be activated, and some are not metabolized at all. Indeed, some harmless chemicals are converted into carcinogens by the liver.

The first-pass effect, mentioned above, occurs because all of the blood from the intestines goes to the liver first (see Figure 1.4). This can be overcome clinically if necessary by giving the drug by a different route (e.g., sublingually or parenterally) or by giving the drug at a higher dose (if 50% is degraded on first pass, give two times as much). A problem with the latter approach is that different people can vary dramatically in their ability to metabolize drugs.

An additional complication that affects dosing is that the concentration of enzymes in the liver is not static. The liver responds to certain drugs by increasing the level of the enzymes that metabolize it. This is called *enzyme induction*. This causes drugs to be broken down faster, resulting in a lower plasma concentration than predicted by the dose given. It also produces metabolic tolerance, whereby a drug has less effect over time as the enzyme that metabolizes it increases.

Cross-tolerance is another potential problem. This is when one drug increases the level of enzymes that break down other drugs. This is a classic drug interaction and can complicate the treatment of a patient who is on several drugs or patients who are using recreational drugs that they don't disclose to their physician.

Finally, some drugs can block the metabolism of other drugs. An example of this is the effect of taking drugs with grapefruit juice. The phytochemicals in grapefruit juice are broken down in the liver by the same enzymes that break down drugs. Grapefruit juice has a high concentration of these phytochemicals, which overwhelms the enzymes in the liver. This causes enzyme inhibition because the liver enzymes are occupied with breaking down the phytochemicals. The result is a dramatic increase in the plasma concentration of a drug, which can lead to a dangerous and even fatal overdose.

Elimination

The main means of eliminating a drug and its metabolites from the body is through the kidneys. Some drugs are secreted into the bile in the liver and eliminated by the gastrointestinal tract, but these are rare. The role of the kidneys is to filter the blood to remove toxins and metabolic wastes. The kidneys receive 20% of the blood from the heart and process the entire blood volume in approximately one hour.

The functional unit of the kidney is the nephron (see Figure 1.11). At the beginning of the nephron is Bowman's capsule. Here, the capillaries of the incoming blood have fenestrations (holes) that allow all dissolved particles to escape the blood. Only particles as large as proteins are held back. Drugs are filtered out, along with salts, glucose, amino acids, and other polar molecules, many of which are needed by the body. In the next segments of the nephron, the descending and ascending loops of Henle, water, salts, and nutrients are reabsorbed and returned to the blood. Polar molecules that aren't specifically reabsorbed (e.g., polar drugs and metabolic wastes such as urea) stay in urine. The dilute urine in the nephron is then emptied into the collecting duct, where water is reabsorbed to concentrate it. This concentration of the urine is controlled here by a hormone called *antidiuretic hormone* (*ADH*), which will be discussed in Chapter 7 on alcohol.

The important mechanism utilized by the kidney is selective reabsorption. Anything polar that isn't actively reabsorbed stays in the urine and is eliminated. In this way, metabolized drugs that are either polar or are made polar by the liver are removed from the blood and excreted in the urine. However, nonpolar drugs can cross membranes of the nephron and blood vessels and diffuse back into the blood. This increases the amount of time they stay in the body.

Drug Clearance

The clearance of a drug from the blood is a product of the functions of the liver and kidneys, or metabolism and elimination. Chemicals that are very polar (e.g., vitamin C) or rapidly

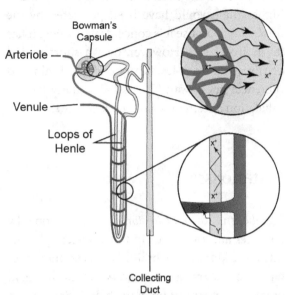

Figure 1.11 In Bowman's capsule of the nephron (upper inset), fenestrations in the capillaries allow all dissolved materials to diffuse out, including polar drugs (X+) and nonpolar drugs (Y). In the ascending and descending loops of Henle (lower inset) nonpolar drugs can diffuse through the cells of the loop and back into the bloodstream while polar drugs are trapped in the loop. They will eventually leave the body in the urine via the collecting duct.

metabolized (e.g., cocaine) are removed from the body quickly. Chemicals that are nonpolar and not well metabolized, such as methamphetamine, last longer in the body.

First-Order Kinetics

Most chemicals, whether removed quickly or slowly, are removed by first-order kinetics (see Figure 1.12A). In first-order elimination, the amount of the drug cleared from the blood per unit of time is dependent on the concentration of the drug in the blood. At a high concentration of the drug, the liver enzymes work faster, and more is removed. As time goes on, there is less drug to be metabolized, and it is eliminated more slowly.

This results in a half-life of drug removal. One *half-life* is the amount of time it takes for half of the drug to be removed from the plasma. After one half-life, 50% of the drug has been removed. After the next half-life passes, half of what is left is removed, leaving 25% in the body. After eight half-lives, more than 99% of the drug has been removed. Because the levels of detection of a drug in the blood or urine are much lower than the levels needed to produce an effect, drugs can be detected long after the effect is gone. This

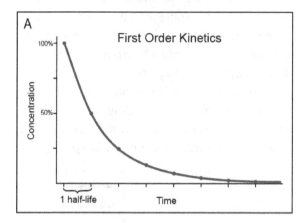

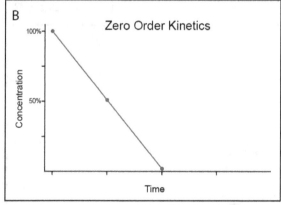

Figure 1.12 A. In first order kinetics, the rate of drug removal is based on its concentration in the blood. For each half-life, half of the drug in the blood is removed. The concentration of drug asymptotically approaches zero; > 99% of it is removed after 8 half-lives. B. In zero order elimination, the amount removed is constant over time.

time is increased if the drug partitions into fatty tissues, as described above.

Zero-Order Kinetics

One important drug that is not eliminated according to first-order kinetics is alcohol. Alcohol is taken in doses much higher than those of other drugs to produce its effect. For example, 2 mg of diazepam (Valium) has about the same effect as 20 grams of alcohol, a ten-thousandfold difference in amount. For this reason, even the lowest dose of ethanol taken recreationally maximizes the capacity of the enzymes that metabolize it. Because the enzymes are working as fast as they can, they eliminate alcohol at a constant rate (see Figure 1.12B). This is called *zero-order kinetics*.

Variables That Affect a Drug's Half-Life

The half-life of a drug can vary dramatically in length between different people. This can be due to a number of factors. For one, liver metabolism can differ. People can inherit slightly different forms of enzymes (isoforms), and levels of enzymes can differ between people. Kidney function, the other important factor in drug clearance, can also vary between people. Body composition (lean body mass), which varies significantly between people, can also affect the distribution of nonpolar drugs. Partitioning into fatty tissue delays removal from the system, and people with more fatty tissue will store more of the drug.

Some physiological variables can help predict differences in pharmacokinetics. Age can affect liver metabolism and kidney function. The elderly and very young have lower function in these important organs and should be given smaller doses. Gender can also have an effect due to differences in body size, body composition, and hormones. Finally, pregnancy adds an additional stress on maternal organs and affects the way drugs are processed.

Time Course of Drug Effect

The amount of time that a drug is in the body, either at an effective dose or lingering in the body afterward, is affected by all four processes of pharmacokinetics. Clinically, these parameters are well established and are accounted for by doctors prescribing the medicine. For recreational drugs, the user may be unaware of the pharmacokinetics or may intuit them based on prior experience. For example, the user may take advantage of the effect of rapid absorption of a drug by IV injection to gain a greater "rush" with the onset of the drug.

Figure 1.13 shows how the route of administration can affect the time course of the drug in the body. The drug used in the hypothetical example is oxycodone. This pharmaceutical can be prescribed in normal, immediate-release tablets, which dissolve in the stomach and release the dose of oxycodone all at once, or extended-release tablets (e.g., OxyContin), which have three to four times higher doses but are compounded to release the oxycodone over twelve hours.

There are three important things to note about this graph. First, once the absorption and distribution of the drug are complete, the clearance from the body occurs at the same rate, no matter what the route of administration was. Metabolism and elimination are constant and determine the half-life of removal of the drug after absorption is complete.

Second, the rate of absorption can affect the peak concentration of the drug, as well as the time to peak and duration in the body. With a very fast to immediate route of absorption, such

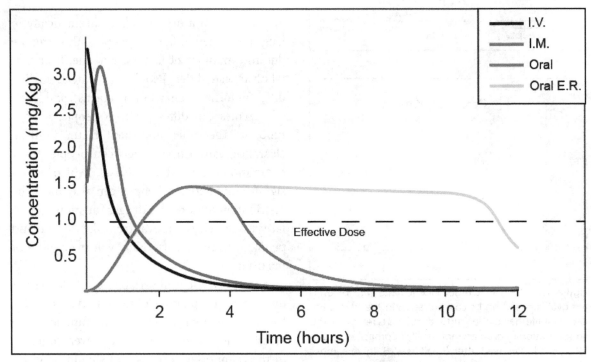

Figure 1.13 Time course of drug effect. The route of administration can greatly affect the peak of the drug and the amount of time that it is in the body. An extended release formulation (Oral E.R.)

as with an IV, the total dose of the drug is in the system immediately, and the drug concentration peaks at its maximum. With a slow means of absorption, such as oral administration, metabolism and elimination are occurring at the same time as absorption. By the time the last of the drug has been absorbed, some of it has been removed from the blood, which reduces the peak. (There are also the effects of bioavailability and the first-pass effect, which will decrease the peak of an orally administered drug.)

Third, note the time course of the extended-release formulation of oxycodone. The onset of effect is the same as the immediate-release oral administration's onset, because they are both taken orally. However, the extended-release oxycodone stays in the effective dose range much longer than the immediate-release version does. The extended-release formulation breaks down slowly during the passage through the small intestine, as described above, and releases the drug as it moves along. But to maintain the drug above this effective dose for this long time period, the amount of drug in the formulation has to be three to four times as high. This is because metabolism and elimination are occurring at a constant rate and continue to remove the drug from the body as it is released. The constant dose level in the center of the curve represents the breakdown of the formulation and release of the drug in balance with its metabolism and elimination.

Summary

Pharmacokinetics is the study of the rate of drugs moving into and out of the body. The pharmacokinetics of a drug can greatly influence the effects of the drug on the individual. There are four processes in pharmacokinetics. Absorption is the movement of the drug across the barriers of the body and into the bloodstream. There are five common means of administering a drug. Oral administration is the slowest, but the easiest and often safest means of administration. It can be variable because of the first-pass effect and bioavailability of the drug. Rectal administration can be used for unconscious or vomiting patients, and it avoids most of the first-pass effects of oral administration. Parenteral administration, or injection, is a very rapid means of administration and the best means to control the dosage of a drug. The three common means of parenteral administration are intravenous, intramuscular, and subcutaneous. Inhalation is the fastest means of administration, but can only be used for volatile drugs. Finally, topical administration involves the drug diffusing across a mucous membrane (e.g., nasal cavity, mouth, or skin). The polarity of the drug is very important in topical administration, in that only nonpolar drugs are able to cross these membranes. Once the drug is in the bloodstream, the process of distribution ensures that all cells experience the same concentration of the drug. One caveat is the brain, which is protected by the blood-brain barrier. Only nonpolar drugs are able to cross this. The drug is removed from the body by the processes of metabolism and elimination. Metabolism, which is performed mainly in the liver, involves enzymes attempting to make the molecule more polar. This can inactivate or activate the drug, but usually makes the drug more water soluble so that it can be excreted by the kidneys into the urine. Metabolism and elimination determine the half-life of the drug in the body, which is usually a first-order process.

Further Reading

Winter, Michael E. *Basic Clinical Pharmacokinetics.* 5th ed. Philadelphia, PA: Lippincott Williams & Williams, 2010.

Oral absorption: Heikkinen, A. T., T. Korjamo, and J. Monkkonen. "Modelling of Drug Disposition Kinetics in *In Vitro* Intestinal Absorption Cell Models." *Basic & Clinical Pharmacology & Toxicology* 106 (2009): 180–8.

Routes of administration: Fattinger, K., N. L. Benowitz, R. T. Jones, and D. Verotta. "Nasal Mucosal versus Gastrointestinal Absorption of Nasally Administered Cocaine." *European Journal of Clinical Pharmacology* 56 (2000): 305–10.

Metabolic differences between populations: Barter, Z. E., G. T. Tucker, and K. R. Yeo. "Differences in Cytochrome P450-Mediated Pharmacokinetics Between Chinese and Caucasian Populations Predicted by Mechanistic Physiologically Based Pharmacokinetic Modelling." *Clinical Pharmacokinetics* 52 (2013): 1085–100.

Variation in elimination: Yuen, G. J. "Altered Pharmacokinetics in the Elderly." *Clinics in Geriatric Medicine* 6 (1990): 257–67.

Extended-release formulation: Cruciani, R. A. "Dose Equivalence of Immediate-Release Hydromorphone and Once-Daily Osmotic-Controlled Extended-Release Hydromorphone: A Randomized, Double-Blind Trial Incorporating a Measure of Assay Sensitivity." *Journal of Pain* 13 (2012): 379–89.

Blood-brain barrier: Voica, V. A. "New Insights on the Consequences of Biotransformation Processes on the Distribution and Pharmacodynamic Profiles of Some Neuropsychotropic Drugs." *European Neuropsychopharmacology* 22 (2012): 319–29.

Test Your Understanding
Multiple-Choice

1. Which of the following is not a function of the polarity of a drug?
   a. its absorption via an intravenous injection
   b. its ability to enter the brain
   c. its transdermal absorption
   d. the ability of the kidneys to excrete it
2. Which means of absorption is the fastest route to the brain?
   a. oral
   b. rectal
   c. inhalation
   d. intravenous
3. In inhalation of a drug, its absorption occurs in the
   a. trachea
   b. bronchi
   c. bronchioles
   d. alveoli
4. The first-pass effect is a barrier to drugs taken by
   a. IM
   b. inhalation
   c. topically
   d. orally
5. The two-compartment model predicts that
   a. nonpolar drugs will partition into the aqueous areas of the body
   b. nonpolar drugs will last longer in the body
   c. polar drugs will be eliminated slowly from the body

      d. polar drugs will have a stronger effect in the brain
6. The induction of enzymes in the liver
      a. can create cross-tolerance, where one drug affects another's concentration
      b. increases the variability of drug dosing
      c. causes drugs to be broken down faster
      d. all of the above
7. Which of the following is not true about a drug's clearance?
      a. it is inhibited by extensive metabolism by the liver
      b. it is usually first-order, with a half-life
      c. it can vary between people based on kidney function
      d. it can be affected by the polarity of the drug
8. The rate of absorption of a drug can affect
      a. the peak concentration of the drug
      b. the duration of the drug in the body
      c. the amount of "rush" produced by the drug
      d. all of the above

Essay Questions

1. Describe the route a drug takes to the brain when it is injected intramuscularly.
2. Explain the role of the kidney and why it relies on the liver for help to perform this role.
3. Some potent opiates, which activate the same receptors as morphine or heroin, are available as over-the-counter medicines that anyone can buy in the drugstore as antidiarrheal medicines. However, they produce no euphoria or sedation like morphine does. Why might this be (based on pharmacokinetic principles)?
4. Two people take the same dose of heroin; one snorts it, and the other swallows the same dose. One person overdoses and is sent to the hospital, and the other is alert enough to call the ambulance. Which one is sent to the hospital and why?
5. Explain why a drug can be detected in the urine days or weeks after the effect of the drug has worn off.

Credit

- Fig. 1.0: Copyright © by Depositphotos / Ziablik.

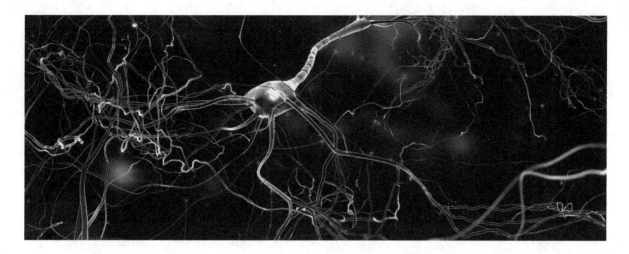

Chapter 2: Pharmacodynamics I

Nerve Cells and the Brain

Most recreational drugs are psychoactive, which is to say that they are taken for their effects on the brain. Peripherally acting drugs, like antacids or antihistamines, are typically not taken just for fun. Psychoactive drugs produce their effects by altering the activity of nerve cells in the brain. So, in order to understand how the drugs work, it is important to understand the normal physiology of nerve cells.

Each nerve cell is a link in a web of hundreds of billions of nerves that together make tens of trillions of connections. The combined activity of all these nerve cells receives stimuli from the outside world through the senses, maintains the "housekeeping" aspects of physiology through the autonomic and hormonal systems (heat rate, breathing, body temperature, etc.), coordinates movement by controlling the skeletal muscles, and creates consciousness.

There are two main types of cells in the brain (excluding blood vessels and blood cells that nourish the brain). These are neurons and glial cells. Neurons receive input (usually chemical but often electrical) from a number of other neurons, add together the input from these sources, and then conduct electrical impulses to other neurons in response to this integration of inputs. Glial cells are mainly support cells for the neurons, providing metabolic support, protecting the brain from toxins, and insulating axons to increase their conduction. This chapter will look at both of these cells and their contributions to brain function.

Neuron Structure

The neuron has a number of important parts (see Figure 2.1). Dendrites extend from the cell body (soma) and branch out to receive information. A neuron can have a single dendrite, many dendrites, or no dendrites at all, as the soma can also directly receive information. Dendrites have tiny extensions called dendritic spines that reach toward the axon bulb of other neurons to form synapses. These spines can be increased or decreased in number by the cell in response to the amount of input the cell receives at each synapse. (This will be important in the discussion of neuroadaptation in Chapter 5.) The dendrite receives chemicals (neurotransmitters) from the axons of other neurons at the synapse, converts this chemical signal into an electrical signal, and relays this signal to the soma. This begins the process of integration.

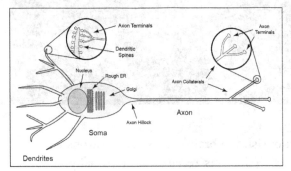

Figure 2.1 Insets represent magnification of the terminals. Axonal bulbs on the left represent on collaterals from a neuron interacting with this dendrite.

The axon is a single long extension of the soma that begins at an area called the axon hillock. The axon splits into collaterals near its end in most neurons, which increases the number of synapses that it forms. The axon receives electrical signals from the soma at the axon hillock and converts this into an action potential that is transmitted to the synaptic terminals (often called terminal buttons or bulbs). The axon bulb releases a neurotransmitter (chemical signal) at a synapse with another neuron. As with the dendritic spines, the number of collaterals and axon bulbs can be increased or decreased based on the amount of neurotransmission occurring. Most axons are wrapped in insulation called myelin (see Figure 2.2), which increases the speed of electrical transmission of the action potentials.

The cell body, or soma, performs the same activities performed by other cells in the body that are necessary to maintain life. It stores the DNA of the genome in its nucleus and accesses

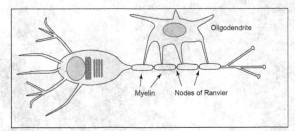

Figure 2.2 The oligodendrite shown has wrapped processes around the axon of the neuron producing a myelin sheath.

this information to produce proteins. Its ribosomes, rough endoplasmic reticulum and Golgi apparatus synthesize the proteins, package them, and ship them to their proper destinations. This maintains the structure and function of the cell. It also has mitochondria that produce energy to run the cell's processes. In addition, the plasma membrane of the soma receives and integrates electrical information directly from synapses and indirectly from dendrites. Each soma can receive information from thousands of synapses. The soma adds together or integrates this information by the process of summation, much like a microprocessor in a computer, and relays it to the axon hillock. If the soma is receiving enough excitatory information, this will stimulate the axon hillock to produce an action potential that will be carried to the axon terminals. There will be much more discussion about this process later in this chapter.

Glial Cells

Glial cells represent about half of the volume of neural tissue in the brain and perform many vital tasks. There are two major types of glial cells: astrocytes and oligodendrites. Astrocytes (named for their star-shaped appearance) provide metabolic support to the neuronal soma; they store glycogen for release as glucose during times of high activity, clear synapses of neurotransmitters (especially glutamate and GABA), and can regulate the extracellular concentration of K^+, which has profound effects on neuronal activity. In addition, astrocytes wrap processes around the capillaries of the brain. In this way they regulate the microcirculation in the brain, ensuring that the neurons receive adequate O_2 and nutrients. Also, this wrapping produces the blood brain barrier discussed in Chapter 1. Polar chemicals are excluded from the brain by this barrier and only nonpolar chemicals can get through.

The main function of oligodendrites is to wrap the axons with insulation called myelin (see Figure 2.2). Myelin is a fatty layer that restricts the electrical activity in the axon so that the action potential skips between the gaps in the myelin. These gaps are call Nodes of Ranvier. The action potential occurs here and then is passed through the myelinated regions to the next node via saltatory conduction (discussed below). This greatly increases the rate that the action potential moves down the axon (10- to 30-fold increase in conduction velocity!).

Membrane Potential

The plasma membranes of excitable cells (like neurons and muscle cells) maintain an electrical potential (voltage) that is used to pass information. The membrane potential is produced by 2 aspects of the membrane: asymmetric distribution of ions and selective permeability of ions.

The extracellular fluid of cells, which is maintained fairly constant by blood flow, is high in sodium (about 145 mM Na^+) and low in potassium (about 4.0 mM K^+). In neurons, the internal concentration of these ions is much different: Na^+ is approximately 12 mM and K^+ is approximately 139 mM. Other ions that are

important are chloride (Cl^-) and calcium (Ca^{2+}), but we will disregard them for now. Sodium and potassium are asymmetrically distributed by the action of the sodium potassium ATPase (NKA, see Figure 2.3). NKA uses the energy of 1 ATP molecule to pump 3 Na^+ out of the cell for every 2 K^+ in. This produces the gradients for Na^+ and K^+ and represents stored chemical energy. Na^+ has a large chemical driving force to enter the cell and K^+ has a large chemical driving force to exit the cell (see Figure 2.3).

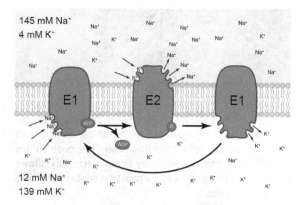

Figure 2.3 The Na^+-K^+ ATPase has 2 states, E1 and E2, which are controlled by phosphorylation. In the E1 state, it binds 3 Na^+ ions and ATP on the inside of the membrane. It then uses the ATP to phosphorylate itself and change to the E2 conformation. In the E2 state it releases the 3 Na^+ on the outside of the membrane and picks up 2 K^+. The enzyme then de-phosphorylates and converts back to the E1 state, releasing K^+ on the inside of the membrane.

The second piece of the puzzle is selective permeability. The plasma membrane is nonpolar, so the charged Na^+ and K^+ are prevented from diffusing directly through the membrane down their chemical gradients. To pass through the membrane they must go through protein channels that span the membrane. These are proteins with many transmembrane segments that align to form a water-filled pore through the membrane (see Figure 2.4). Channels also have a

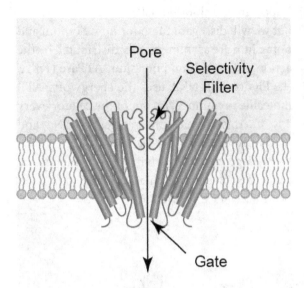

Figure 2.4 Most ion channels have multiple transmembrane domains (represented by cylinders) arranged to produce a water filled pore in the center. The pore includes domains that form a selectivity filter, which only allows one type of ion through, and a gate that controls whether the ions can pass.

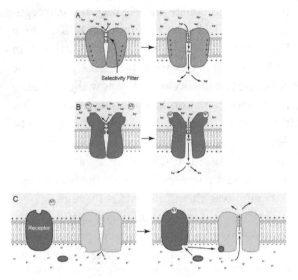

Figure 2.5 There are 3 main ways that ion channels are gated: by the voltage of the membrane (A), by binding of a neurotransmitter (NT) to the extracellular domains (B), or by a metabolic process activated by a neurotransmitter binding to a receptor (C).

selectivity filter in the pore; each type of channel is selective for one ion. There are Na^+ channels, K^+ channels, Ca^{2+} channels, and Cl^- channels to conduct each of these ions.

Most channels are regulated (gated) in some manner. There are three main ways that channels are regulated (see Figure 2.5). Voltage dependent channels open and close based on the voltage of the membrane. Usually these are closed at resting membrane potentials and open when the membrane depolarizes. Ligand gated channels are regulated by the binding of a neurotransmitter to the external domains of the channel (in Chapter 3 these will be called ionotropic receptors). There are also metabolically activated channels that are opened and closed by some enzymatic process (in Chapter 3 these will be called metabotropic receptors). There are

other ways that ion channels can be gated but these are the most common.

At any moment, the membrane will have one ion that is most permeable. This is because it has the most channels open. For example, in a neuron at rest there are some unregulated K^+ channels that allow K^+ to leave the cell (see Figure 2.6). These are called K^+ leak channels and the K^+ ions that leak out of the cell leave behind negative charges (mainly on proteins and amino acids). As a result, this leak produces an electrical potential (voltage) across the membrane. An electrode poked into the cell would measure a negative voltage on the inside of the membrane, compared to the outside of the membrane. This is the membrane potential (Vm). For the movement of Na^+, the opposite would happen; if Na^+ channels open and Na^+ is allowed to move through the membrane freely, its chemical driving force would cause it to move into the cell, making the inside of the membrane more positive.

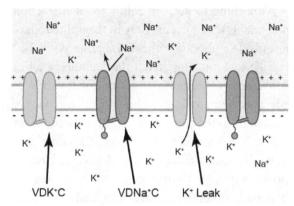

Figure 2.6 At rest, there is a K⁺ leak out of the cell. This loss of K+ leaves negative charges behind, which leaves the inside of the membrane negative.

Resting Membrane Potential

At rest, most channels in the neuron's membrane are closed. However, there is a significant leak of K^+ out of the cell. There is also a Na^+ leak into the cell, but the K^+ leak is much greater, so it is the most permeable ion. For this reason, at rest the inside of the membrane is negative, somewhere around −70 mV. If the voltage of the membrane moves in the positive direction, this is called depolarization. If the membrane moves more negative, this is called hyperpolarization. Depolarizing the membrane opens the voltage dependent ion channels mentioned above. This is the key to understanding how the membrane potential changes during an action potential.

An Action Potential

An action potential (AP) is the controlled opening and closing of voltage dependent ion channels, which changes the membrane voltage. APs are the result of the integration of inputs received by the soma at synapses and is the way that the neuron sends information to the next neuron in the network. APs only occur in the axons of neurons. They start at the axon hillock and stop when they reach the axon bulbs.

Electrical activity in the soma spreads passively to the axon hillock, depolarizing it. This depolarizing stimulus from the soma initiates the AP by activating voltage dependent sodium channels (VDNa⁺C). VDNa⁺Cs (see Figure 2.7) can be in one of 3 different conformational states. At the resting membrane potential, the VDNa⁺C is in the "closed" state. In this state the voltage gate blocks the pore and no Na^+ can enter the cell. The channel is in this state when the membrane is at rest (-70 mV). A depolarizing stimulus causes the voltage gate to shift, opening the pore. The VDNa⁺C is then in the "open" state. Na^+ passes through the channel in this state causing depolarization of the membrane. After a brief passage of time (1-3 ms), an inactivating particle that is part of the channel blocks the pore. The VDNa⁺C is then in the "inactive" state and Na^+ cannot pass. To go back to the closed state, the membrane has to repolarize back to the resting

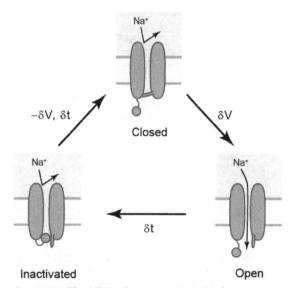

Figure 2.7 The VDNa⁺C can exist in one of three states: closed (or available), open, or inactivated. This depends on the voltage of the membrane.

Vm; the VDNa+Cs then go back to the closed state over a period of a few milliseconds and are "available" to open again.

The first phase of the AP occurs when the VDNa+Cs in the axon hillock are stimulated by depolarization from the soma to go from the closed to the open state (see Figure 2.8). This greatly increases the permeability of the membrane to Na+ and it rushes into the cell, depolarizing it to approximately +40 mV. Slightly before the peak of the action potential, voltage dependent K+ channels (VDK+Cs), which operate similar to VDNa+Cs, go from the closed to the open state. At the same time, the VDNa+Cs are going from open to inactivated. Because of the K+ leaving the cell, the membrane potential goes back to and past the original Vm; it hyperpolarizes to approximately –80 mV. This is called the undershoot. At this point, the VDK+Cs close again, bringing the membrane potential back to resting (–70 mV), and the VDNa+Cs go from the inactivated state back to the closed state. The membrane is now ready to initiate another AP.

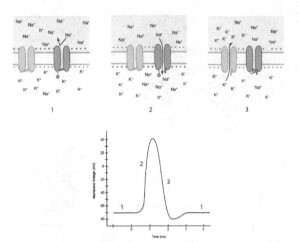

Figure 2.8 The diagrams at the top show the states of the VDNa+C and VDK+C at rest, during the rising phase of the AP (depolarization), and during the repolarization of the axon. The graph below shows how these changes in channel state affect the membrane voltage, producing the action potential.

One thing to keep in mind about the action potential is that it occurs only in the limited space just inside and outside the membrane. While Na+ and K+ ions moving across the membrane affect the voltage on the membrane, they have very little effect on the overall intracellular concentrations of these ions in the short term. Long term, the NKA is always active and reestablishes their concentrations. However, if the activity of NKA is blocked (for example, by the drug digitalis) the concentration gradients of the ions will eventually run down and the neuron will lose its membrane potential.

The Threshold and All-or-Nothing APs

In the first phase of the AP, the depolarizing stimulus from the soma opens the VDNa+Cs. However, not every depolarization causes an action potential to initiate. If the depolarization is weak (just a few mV) it will open only a few VDNa+Cs. The Na+ entry through these channels will further depolarize the axon hillock. However, there is still a K+ leak out of the cell that can counteract this depolarization. If the K+ leak is stronger than the depolarization, the axon hillock goes back to resting Vm and no AP is generated. If, however, enough VDNa+Cs are opened by the depolarization that the Na+ entering outmatches the K+ leak, this causes more VDNa+Cs to open, further depolarizing the membrane. This depolarization causes more VDNa+Cs to open, which allows more Na+ entry and more VDNa+C opening. This positive feedback cycle opens all the VDNa+Cs. At this point the action potential peaks and begins to propagate down the axon (discussed below).

The scenario above results in a threshold for initiation of an action potential (see Figure 2.9). Any depolarization below this threshold and the axon hillock repolarizes due to the K+ leak. Any depolarization above this threshold and all the VDNa+Cs open, initiating an AP. The threshold for AP initiation in mammalian neurons is approximately -50 mV.

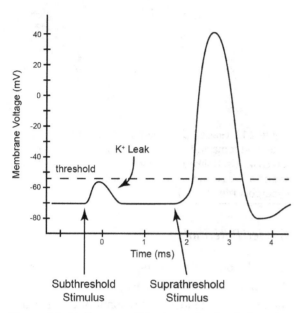

Figure 2.9 At the axon hillock, a stimulus below the threshold potential (subthreshold) will be counteracted by the K+ leak and return to the resting Vm. A superthreshold stimulus surpasses the threshold voltage, opens all of the VDNa+C, and generates an AP.

This threshold makes AP initiation an all-or-nothing event. Either the threshold is crossed and AP is initiated or no AP starts. If an AP is initiated, all VDNa+Cs open and it is at maximum intensity. Therefore, there are no strong or weak APs; they are all the same magnitude. Increasing the stimulus from the soma to the axon hillock causes an increased *frequency* of APs in the axon (i.e., a new one initiates as soon as the membrane repolarizes), not stronger APs.

Passive Spread of Depolarization and AP Propagation

When one area or patch of membrane is depolarized, this voltage spreads passively (i.e., without opening of channels) across the membrane. This

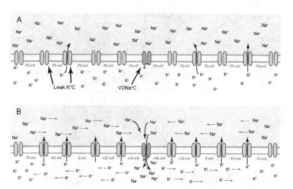

Figure 2.10 A. The leak of K+ out of the cell maintains the resting membrane potential around -70 mV. B. When voltage dependent Na+ channels (VDNa+C) open, Na+ floods into the cell. This creates a current of K+ movement away from the site due to charge repulsion, spreading the depolarization along the membrane. The voltage decreases with distance from the site due to the K+ leak channels.

is true in the membrane of the dendrites and soma (discussed below) as well as the axon. This passive spread of depolarization decreases in magnitude with distance away from the source of depolarization due to the K+ leak out of the cell (see Figure 2.10).

The passive spread of depolarization causes the AP to move from the axon hillock to the axon bubs as a wave of depolarization and repolarization. You can think of this movement as passing from one patch of membrane to the next (see Figure 2.11). As one patch of membrane depolarizes, the depolarization passively spreads to the next patch. This opens the VDNa+Cs there causing this patch to depolarize. As the second patch is depolarizing, the first patch is repolarizing due to activation of the VDK+Cs, and the depolarization from the second patch spreads to the third patch, initiating an AP there. In this way, the AP passes down the axon like dominoes falling down (depolarizing) and then resetting themselves (repolarizing).

In myelinated neurons this occurs much faster. This is because the myelination insulates

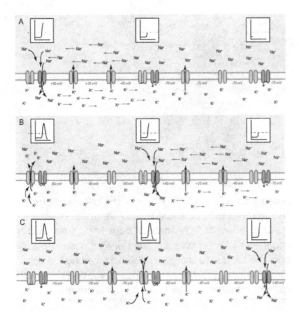

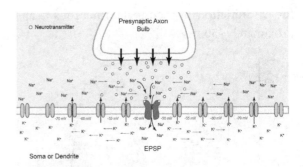

Figure 2.13 Graded potentials are produced in the dendrites and soma and are due to the opening ligand gated ion channels. Unlike APs, they vary in magnitude, being strong or weak, and can be either depolarizing (EPSPs) or hyperpolarizing (IPSPs).

Figure 2.11 Depolarization produced by an AP in one patch of the membrane (A, left) is passively conducted to the next adjacent patch (A, middle). This opens VDNa$^+$Cs in this patch, generating an action potential here (B). The depolarization in B is relayed passively to the next patch (right), which then initiates an action potential (C). The generation of the action potential in each patch is depicted in the graphs above.

Graded Potentials

Graded potentials (see Figure 2.13) differ from APs in several important ways. First, they occur mainly in the dendrites and soma of the neuron. Second, they are produced by neurotransmitters (NTs) released at synapses activating ligand-gated channels. Finally, these potentials are not all-or-nothing; instead they vary in magnitude, being strong or weak and either depolarizing or hyperpolarizing.

Dendrites and the soma have no voltage dependent channels. Graded potentials produced there are due to opening ligand-gated ion channels (which will be discussed in more detail in the next chapter). Ions passing through these channels affect the membrane potential transiently, lasting only as long as the NT is present, which is very brief. When the NT is cleared from the synapse, the ligand-gated channel closes again and the K$^+$ leak re-establishes the resting potential.

Each type of ligand-gated ion channel passes only one type of ion, either Na$^+$, K$^+$, or Cl$^-$. The response of the membrane depends on which of these ions is passing through. If it is a Na$^+$ channel, the membrane depolarizes. Since this takes the cell closer to an AP, this change in potential is called

the axon in the area between the nodes. This eliminates the K$^+$ leak and allows the passive spread of depolarization to go much further (see Figure 2.12). This is called saltatory conduction and it greatly increases the speed of conduction of the AP down the axon.

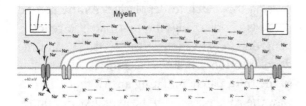

Figure 2.12 Depolarization in one node of Ranvier is conducted, slightly diminished, to the next node via saltatory conduction. This passive spread of depolarization goes much further than in unmyelinated neurons, resulting in a faster conduction speed of the AP.

an Excitatory Postsynaptic Potential (EPSP). If the ion passing through is either Cl⁻ entering or K⁺ leaving, the membrane becomes more negative or hyperpolarized from the resting potential. Since this takes the cell further away from an AP, this is called an Inhibitory Postsynaptic Potential (IPSP).

The actual response (IPSP or EPSP) depends which neurotransmitter is released at the synapse and which receptors are present. Each axon synapsing with a neuron only releases one type of neurotransmitter and the receptor will be specific for it. As such, each synapse will be either excitatory or inhibitory.

Integration by Nerve Cells

The dendrites and soma of a neuron are acted on by axon bulbs from many other neurons. Some of these are excitatory (producing EPSPs) and some are inhibitory (producing IPSPs). When one of these postsynaptic potentials is produced it spreads passively away from the site of origin, as described above, diminishing with distance from the site of origin. If strong enough, its effect can be felt at the axon hillock, which is the site of AP initiation (see Figure 2.14A).

EPSPs depolarize the membrane potential, bringing the axon hillock closer to the threshold for generation of an AP. One EPSP alone is not enough to produce an AP. Several must be added together to reach the threshold; this process is called summation. If several EPSPs are produced close together in time by one synapse, these add together to depolarize the membrane to a greater extent. This is called temporal summation. If two synapses near each other on the same neuron produce EPSPs at the same time, these also add together. This is called spatial summation (see Figure 2.14B). Inhibitory inputs (IPSPs) will also

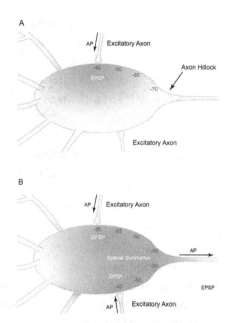

Figure 2.14 A. An excitatory neuron produces and EPSP in the soma of a neuron. This depolarization spreads passively across the membrane, diminishing with distance from the source. B. Depolarization from two excitatory neurons are added together to create a greater depolarization of the membrane. This can surpass the threshold for AP initiation in the axon hillock.

be summed with the excitatory inputs, subtracting from their depolarizing influence.

All of the inputs, EPSPs and IPSPs, are summed in the membrane of the soma and the result affects the membrane potential at the axon hillock. When excitatory inputs exceed the inhibitory inputs, the membrane potential exceeds the threshold for AP initiation at the axon hillock and an AP starts down the axon. When inhibitory inputs exceed the excitatory inputs, the threshold will not be met and the axon will be quiet. If the number of EPSPs greatly exceed the number of IPSPs, the result is an increased frequency AP initiation in the axon hillock. Therefore, when the neuron receives more stimulatory input, it produces more AP output. It then releases more NT in the synapses that it makes with other neurons (see Table 2.1).

Table 2.1: Summation
$\uparrow$ EPSPs in dendrites & soma $\rightarrow$ $\uparrow$ depolarization in cell body & axon hillock $\rightarrow$ $\uparrow$ frequency of APs in axon $\rightarrow$ $\uparrow$ NT release by axon bulbs of this neuron $\uparrow$ IPSPs input in dendrites $\rightarrow$ $\downarrow$ depolarization cell body & axon hillock$\rightarrow$ $\downarrow$ frequency of APs in axon $\rightarrow$ $\downarrow$ NT release by axon bulbs

In this way, the soma of a neuron in one part of the brain receives information from the axons of neurons in other parts of the brain. It adds together all of these inputs to determine the frequency of APs to send down its axon. This axon then goes to another part of the brain and relays this information to neurons there, which similarly add up their inputs. Each neuron is a link in the chain and the sum total of the information processing is the function of the brain.

which depolarizes it, followed by the inactivation of the VDNa$^+$Cs and opening of the VDK$^+$Cs, which repolarizes the membrane. Once an AP occurs in the axon hillock, passive spread of the depolarization opens VDNa$^+$Cs further down the axon causing AP generation there and propagation of the AP down the axon. The AP will travel down the axon until it reaches the axon bulbs. There it causes the release of neurotransmitter, which is the topic of the next chapter.

Summary

Recreational drugs are psychoactive, producing their effects by modifying the function of neurons in the brain. Neurons have dendrites that receive chemical information in the form of neurotransmitters at synapses. They convert this to electrical information (depolarization or hyperpolarization) and relay it to the soma, which can also receive chemical information at synapses. Neurotransmitters at the synapses produce graded potentials, small changes in the membrane potential that can be depolarizing (EPSPs, caused by Na$^+$ entering) or hyperpolarizing (IPSPs, caused by Cl$^-$ entering or K$^+$ leaving). The soma adds together the EPSPs and IPSPs and relays this voltage to the axon hillock. If the soma receives enough EPSPs, it will drop the voltage at the axon hillock below the threshold for generating an AP. An AP is the rapid opening of all of the VDNa$^+$Cs in the membrane,

Further Reading

Myelinated neurons: Arancibia-Caracamo, I.L., and Atwell, D. (2014) "The node of Ranvier in CNS pathology, Acta Neuropathol. 2014; 128(2): 161–175.

Glial cells: Barres, B.A. (2008) The mystery and magic of glia: A perspective on their roles in health and disease. Neuron 60: 430–440

Channel structure/function: Tombola, F., Pathak, M.M., and Isacoff, E.Y. (2006) How Does Voltage Open an Ion Channel? Annual Review of Cell and Developmental Biology 22: 23–52

AP generation: Suart, G., Spruston, N., Sakmann, B., and Hausser, M. (1997) Trends in Neurosciences, 20: 125–131

Levitan, I.B., and Kaczmarek, L.K. (2015) The Neuron, Cell and Molecular Biology Fourth Edition, Oxford University Press, New York, NY, USA

Test Your Understanding

Multiple Choice

1. Which part of the neuron carries information away from the cell?
   a. the soma
   b. the axon
   c. the dendrite
   d. the myelination

2. Which cells wrap around capillaries to produce the blood brain barrier?
   a. astrocytes
   b. oligodendrites
   c. Schwann cells
   d. all of the above

3. The channels that are most important for setting the resting Vm are
   a. VDNa$^+$Cs
   b. VDK$^+$Cs
   c. leak K$^+$ channels
   d. ligand-gated channels

4. The channels that are most important for repolarizing the membrane after and AP are
   a. VDNa$^+$Cs
   b. VDK$^+$Cs
   c. leak K$^+$ channels
   d. ligand-gated channels

5. When the membrane is repolarizing, the VDNa$^+$Cs are in the _____ state.
   a. open
   b. closed
   c. inactivated
   d. repolarized

6. The passive spread of depolarization on the membrane is diminished with distance due to
   a. the VDK$^+$Cs
   b. the resistance of the membrane
   c. the myelination on the axon
   d. the leak K$^+$ channels

7. In what way are graded potentials similar to APs?
   a. they occur mainly in the dendrites and soma of the neuron
   b. they are produced by ion channels that are selective for one ion
   c. they are produced by neurotransmitters
   d. they vary in magnitude, being strong or weak and either depolarizing or hyperpolarizing

8. Opening of an ion channel that allowed Cl$^-$ entry would result in
   a. an IPSP
   b. an EPSP
   c. an AP
   d. none of the above

Essay Questions

1. How are the concentrations of Na$^+$ and K$^+$ different inside and outside of the cell? How is this used to produce an action potential?

2. What is an EPSP? What is an IPSP? How do neurotransmitters produce these in the post-synaptic membrane?

3. Local anesthetics, like lidocaine, block VDNa$^+$Cs. Why would this make them effective as local anesthetics?

4. Why are action potentials all-or-nothing?

5. The drug Valium (diazepam) increases Cl$^-$ current in neurons. What effect will this have on the frequency of APs in a neuron? Explain in terms of summation and integration in the soma.

Credit

- Fig. 2.0: Copyright © by Depositphotos / whitehoune.

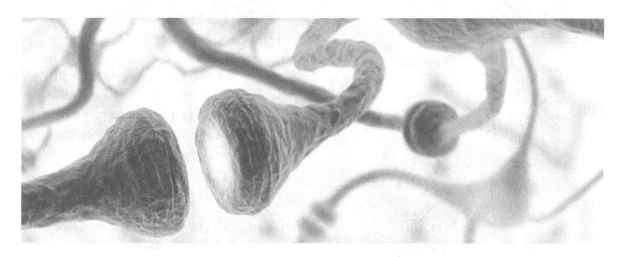

Chapter 3:
Pharmacodynamics II

Introduction

The *synaptic cleft* is a minute gap between communicating neurons. Chemicals, called *neurotransmitters (NTs)*, are released from one side and received by the other. This is how information is passed from one neuron to the next. The understanding of this process is vital to understanding the pharmacology of psychoactive drugs. Most drugs produce their effects by modulating this transmission in some way, either by stimulating it, blocking it, or mimicking it. In this chapter we will discuss the mechanism of synaptic transmission in detail and then how drugs affect it.

Synapses

The synapse can be divided into two sides: (1) the *presynaptic side*, which consists of an axon bulb (or axon terminal), which releases the NT, and (2) the *postsynaptic side*, which receives it.

Synapses can occur between an axon and a dendrite, a soma, or the axon bulb of another neuron (see Figure 3.1). Axodendritic and axosomatic synapses affect the membrane potential of the receiving neuron, while the axoaxonic synapses affect the amount of NTs released by the receiving axon bulb.

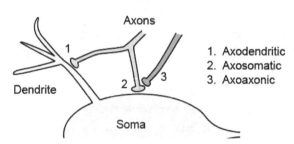

Figure 3.1 Synapses can occur between an axon bulb and a dendrite (1, axodendritic), the soma (2, axosomatic), or an axon bulb (2, axoaxonic) of another neuron.

The Presynaptic Axon Bulbs

The axon bulbs are at the end of the axons. Axons typically split into collaterals, so that each axon has many bulbs and the number of bulbs can be increased or decreased by the neuron. Several processes occur inside the axon bulb to support its function of releasing NTs (see Figure 3.2). Proteins and lipids needed for these processes

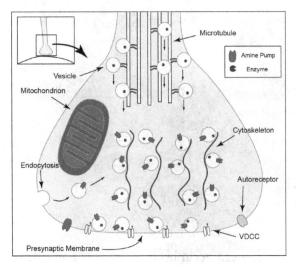

Figure 3.2 Vesicles are transported to the axon bulb via microtubules in the center of the axon. These vesicles then synthesize and accumulate neurotransmitters (NT) and are stored in rows leading to the presynaptic membrane, closely associated with voltage dependent calcium channels (VDCCs). Mitochondria in the axon bulb provide energy for its function. Endocytosis regenerates vesicles after fusion of the vesicles during NT release. Presynaptic autoreceptors provide feedback that regulates NT release.

are transported from the soma down the axon in vesicles that move along a track of microtubules. Mitochondria, also transported to the axon terminals on microtubules, perform the metabolic reactions necessary to provide energy (in the form of ATP) that is used to maintain the function of the bulb.

Vesicles are small, spherical, lipid bilayer sacs. They accumulate in the bulb and are attached to the cytoskeleton. The cytoskeleton holds them in place and moves them into position at the plasma membrane of the synapse. The vesicles have energy-driven pumps that cause them to collect free NTs and precursor molecules for NT production from the cytoplasm. Inside the vesicles there are enzymes that convert precursor molecules into NTs. Thus, the vesicles synthesize, accumulate, and store NTs. Axon bulbs that release peptide NTs, such as endorphins, are

an exception to this. Peptides, like all proteins, are made in the soma.

Vesicles are stored in rows leading to the presynaptic membrane. The most forward set of vesicles attaches to proteins in the membrane in close proximity to voltage-dependent calcium channels (VDCCs) and are primed for release.

Neurotransmitter Release

VDCCs play an important role in the process of NT release. These are channels similar to voltage-dependent sodium channels (see Chapter 2), except that when open they allow Ca^{2+} to enter the cell. There is a large chemical gradient for Ca^{2+} that causes it to flood into the cell when the channels are open (Ca^{2+} is approximately 2 millimolar outside and 0.2 micromolar inside). This gradient is maintained by an enzyme in the plasma membrane similar to sodium potassium ATPase called the Ca^{2+}ATPase (not shown in Figure 3.3).

The process of NT release begins when an action potential (AP) comes down the axon and reaches the axon terminal (see Figure 3.3). The depolarization produced by the AP opens the VDCCs and Ca^{2+} floods into the terminal. Ca^{2+} activates the cytoskeletal proteins that control

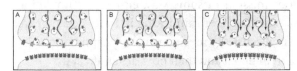

Figure 3.3 A. The axon bulb at rest prepares to release NT by docking vesicles to the presynaptic membrane. B. When the action potential in the axon reaches the presynaptic membrane, the depolarization opens VDCCs and Ca^{2+} floods into the axon bulb. C. Ca^{2+} causes the front row of vesicles to fuse with the presynaptic membrane, spilling their NT into the synapse. The NT activates receptors on the postsynaptic membrane, causing a change in its membrane potential. Vesicles behind the first row move forward, preparing the axon bulb for the next action potential.

the vesicles and causes the front row of vesicles to fuse with the plasma membrane. Fusing causes the release of NTs into the synaptic cleft, and the following rows of vesicles move forward and prepare for the next AP. NT fills the synaptic cleft, diffusing across the gap and interacting with the receptors on the postsynaptic membrane. This results in a change in the membrane potential of the postsynaptic membrane (discussed below).

Autoreceptors

NTs also interact with *autoreceptors*. These are receptors on the presynaptic membrane that are activated by the NT. These receptors serve a role in feedback inhibition. They respond to the NT by inhibiting the VDCCs, preventing further release of NT (see Figure 3.4). This is important feedback for modulating neurotransmission,

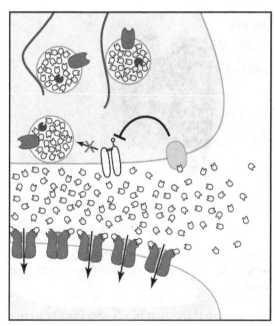

Figure 3.4 Autoreceptors. Autoreceptors on the presynaptic membrane are activated by the released NT. These receptors causes feedback inhibition of the VDCCs, decreasing the amount of Ca^{2+} entry and NT released on subsequent APs.

so that postsynaptic receptors do not become overstimulated and presynaptic axon bulbs do not empty of NT unnecessarily.

Neurotransmitter Removal

After the NT is released, it must be cleared from the synapse to terminate the signal. There are three main ways this is done; the mechanism involved depends on the NT. Many NTs (e.g., dopamine, norepinephrine, and serotonin) are removed from the synapse by a pump on the presynaptic membrane (see Figure 3.5A). This is called the *reuptake pump* or *amine pump*. This pump uses the energy stored in the Na^+ gradient to take the NT from the extracellular fluid and transport it into the cytosol of the axon terminal. In the cytosol, the NT is either recycled into another vesicle or broken down by the mitochondria.

In a second mechanism, other NTs (e.g., glycine and GABA) are cleared from the synapse by astrocytes, which are a type of glial cell. In this mechanism, the NT diffuses out of the synapse, and these helper cells take it up and clear it away (see Figure 3.5B). Often, the astrocyte will then recycle the NT or its metabolic products back into the releasing axonal bulb.

The third mechanism is a special method used by only one NT, acetylcholine. Acetylcholine is broken down in the synapse by the enzyme acetylcholinesterase (see Figure 3.5C). The breakdown products, acetate and choline, are taken up by the presynaptic membrane and reassembled into acetylcholine in the vesicles.

Another important process for maintaining the homeostasis of the axon terminal is endocytosis of the membrane. The fusion of vesicles during NT release adds lipids to the presynaptic membrane. Over time this would lead to a larger and larger presynaptic membrane and a lack of vesicles to store and release NTs. Membrane is

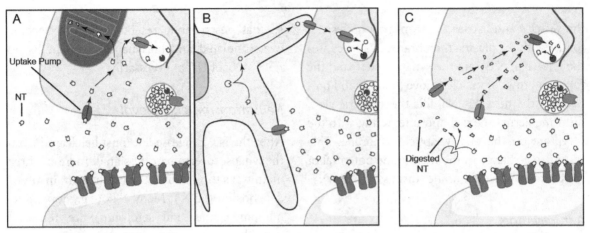

Figure 3.5 A. The most common mechanism of NT removal is via a reuptake pump. This brings the NT back into the axon bulb to either be recycled and re-released or metabolized by the mitochondria. B. Astrocytes clear synapses of some NTs, often recycling the NT back to the releasing axon bulb. C. Acetylcholine is removed from the synapse by acetylcholinesterase degradation. The breakdown products, acetate and choline, are taken up by the presynaptic membrane and resynthesized into acetylcholine.

brought back into the axon bulb by endocytosis to resupply vesicles for NT release and maintain the area of the presynaptic membrane (see Figure 3.2).

The Postsynaptic Membrane

When the NT diffuses across the synapse, it interacts with receptors on the postsynaptic membrane. *Receptors* are transmembrane proteins that bind to the NT on the extracellular side of the membrane and relay this information to the intracellular side. Note that the NT does not enter the cell; the receptor bridges the plasma membrane and relays the information of its presence to the cytosol.

Receptor Structure

There are three domains on a receptor that are important to its function (see Figure 3.6). The ligand binding site is exposed on the extracellular side of the membrane; it reversibly binds the NT.

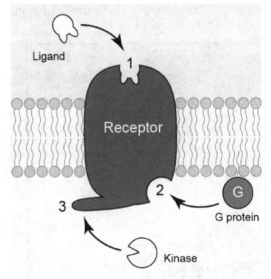

Figure 3.6 A receptor has 3 functional domains: the ligand binding domain (1), the activation domain (2), and the regulation domain (3).

A *ligand* is anything that binds specifically to the binding site. It could be an endogenous NT or a drug molecule. The NT binds to this site very tightly and specifically. The specificity of the interaction, like a key in a lock, is because the amino acids in the binding site have functional groups that are very specific for the structure of the NT. While the NT is very specific for the receptor, some drugs are less so. Less specific drugs will bind to several different types of receptors and can produce side effects. For example, antihistamines are designed to bind to and block histamine receptors. However, they also block some acetylcholine receptors, leading to drowsiness.

The tightness of the drug-receptor interaction is called its *affinity*. The binding of the drug to the receptor is a temporary bond; the drug binds to and then jumps off the receptor, to be replaced by another drug molecule if another is available. How long the drug stays on the receptor before it jumps off is its affinity. This determines the potency of the drug, which is the concentration at which the effect is seen. This relates to the effective dose of the drug. It takes less of a high-affinity drug to produce an effect because it stays on the receptor longer. Note that this does not relate to how powerful the effect of the drug is, only what dose is needed to see the effect.

The second domain on the receptor is the *activation site*. This domain interacts with other cellular proteins when the NT is bound to the receptor. The binding of the NT to the receptor causes a change in the receptor's shape. This change in conformation causes activation of the receptor and allows it to interact with an intracellular protein, activating it. This begins a chain reaction that causes a change in cellular physiology. In the case of NTs, this is either the production of a second messenger or the activation of an ion channel (more on this below in ionotropic receptors and metabotropic receptors). The result is movement of Na^+, K^+, Ca^{2+}, or Cl^- ions across the membrane and the production of graded potentials (discussed in Chapter 2).

When a drug binds to the receptor, there are two possible results. If the drug binds to the receptor and activates it, as the NT does, it mimics the effect of the NT. This type of drug is called is an *agonist*. The drug could also bind to the receptor but not activate it. This drug has no effect on its own, but it blocks the endogenous NT from binding to the receptor, keeping the receptor in the inactive state. This is called an *antagonist* because it blocks the effect of the agonist (NT in this case).

The third site is the *regulatory site*. It is responsible for feedback regulation of the receptor. In addition to producing an effect on the membrane potential, activation of the receptor also turns on a feedback pathway. Second messengers activate kinases that phosphorylate the receptor (i.e., add a phosphate group), causing a decrease in its activity. Similar to autoreceptors, this feedback mechanism protects the cell from overstimulation, but also causes drugs to lose their effect over time. This will be discussed more in the section on receptor regulation below.

Ionotropic Receptors

There are two types of receptors that affect the movement of ions across the membrane, ionotropic and metabotropic receptors. *Ionotropic receptors* are ligand-gated channels (mentioned in Chapter 2). Binding of the NT to this type of receptor opens the channel directly. These represent the minority of types of receptors in the brain (only four), but they produce the majority of neurotransmission in the brain (~90% of NT activity). In the mechanism of this type of receptor, two molecules of the NT bind to the receptor. This causes it to change conformation and open, allowing ions to enter the cell (see Figure 2.5B). This simple mechanism of action produces very fast neurotransmission.

Ionotropic receptors can be linked to either EPSPs or IPSPs. Receptors that respond to the NT glutamate (NMDA and AMPA receptors) are

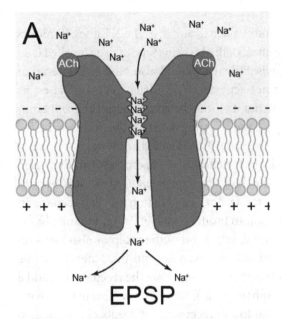
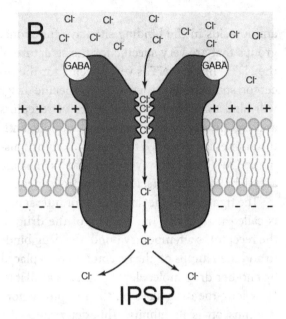

Figure 3.7 A. The binding of 2 molecules of acetylcholine to a nicotinic receptor causes it to open, allowing Na⁺ to enter and producing an EPSP. B. The binding of 2 molecules of GABA to the GABA receptor causes it to open, allowing Cl⁻ to enter and producing an IPSP.

Na⁺ channels, as are one class of receptors that respond to acetylcholine (nicotinic receptors). Activation of these receptors allows Na⁺ to enter the cell, which produces an EPSP, depolarizing the membrane (see Figure 3.7A). Receptors that respond to gamma-aminobutyric acid (GABA) or glycine are Cl⁻ channels. Activation of these receptors allows Cl⁻ to enter the cell, which produces an IPSP, hyperpolarizing the membrane (see Figure 3.7B).

Metabotropic Receptors

The other type of receptors, *metabotropic receptors*, are more complex and indirectly activate ion channels. They represent only a small amount of the activity in the brain (~10%) but have the greatest number of different receptors (hundreds). One way to look at the difference between ionotropic and metabotropic receptors is that while ionotropic receptors drive most of the activity in the brain, metabotropic receptors modulate this activity.

Most metabotropic receptors span the membrane seven times and are called *seven-transmembrane receptors* (*7-TMRs*; see Figure 3.8). They produce effects through intermediary G proteins (and, thus, can also be called *G-protein coupled receptors [GPCRs]*). *G-proteins* are small proteins associated with the membrane that are turned on by the activated receptor and automatically turn themselves off. They link the activated receptor to an effector that produces the effects seen with the NT. Neurotransmitters that use this type of pathway include dopamine, norepinephrine, serotonin, endorphins, and a second class of acetylcholine receptors (muscarinic receptors).

One example of a metabotropic mechanism is when a NT stimulates the production of the second messenger cyclic adenosine monophosphate (cAMP; see Figure 3.9A). This mechanism is common in axon bulbs; it modulates the amount

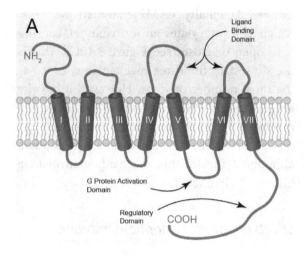

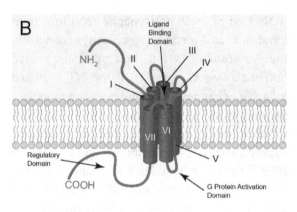

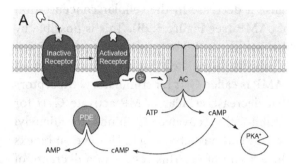

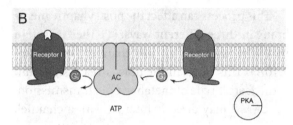

Figure 3.9 A. Activation of receptors linked to increasing cAMP starts a chain reaction leading to the activation of protein kinase A (PKA). The activated receptor activates the G-protein Gs, which activates adenylyl cyclase (AC). AC produces cAMP from ATP, which, in turn, activates PKA. cAMP is broken down by phosphodiesterase (PDE). B. Other receptors are linked to inhibition of AC. Receptor II activates a different isoform of the G-protein, Gi, which binds to and inhibits AC. This blocks the action of Gs.

Figure 3.8 A. 7 TMRs have 7 nonpolar helical segments that span the membrane, an external amino terminus and an internal carboxy terminus (shown in an expanded view). The primary ligand binding portions are on the external loops between transmembrane segments IV and V and segments V and VI. The activation domain is in the internal loop between transmembrane segments V and VI. The regulatory domain is in the carboxy terminal segment. B. The 3 dimensional structure groups the transmembrane segments together.

of NTs released by controlling the VDCC. (This will be central to the effects of many recreational drugs.) The binding of the NT to the receptor causes its activation, which allows it to interact with a G-protein. The G-protein is activated, and it in turn activates the enzyme adenylyl cyclase (AC). AC converts ATP into cAMP, which is the second messenger. cAMP activates a kinase called protein kinase A (PKA). PKA uses ATP to add phosphate to proteins, either activating or inhibiting them. After the NT is removed from the synapse, the second messenger is then removed by the enzyme phosphodiesterase (PDE), which hydrolyses cAMP into AMP. (This is only one example of a signal transduction pathway. Other pathways are important as well but are not included here.)

Some receptors, especially presynaptic autoreceptors, also work through the cAMP second messenger system. However, these receptors cause a decrease in the cellular concentration of cAMP (see Figure 3.9B). This is possible by the use of an isoform of the G-protein. The G-protein associated with the activation of cAMP is called G_s (*s* for stimulatory). Receptors that decrease cellular cAMP activate G_i (*i* for inhibitory). Activated G_i binds to adenylyl cyclase without activating it. However, it blocks the activity of G_s. This results in a decrease of cAMP in the cell.

This process can affect the postsynaptic membrane in three different ways: (1) The G-protein may directly open an ion channel (see Figure 3.10A). This skips all the downstream steps and is the fastest type of metabotropic transmission. (2) cAMP may directly interact with a channel, opening or closing it (see Figure 3.10B). This requires one more step, and is therefore a little slower. (3) Finally, cAMP may activate PKA, which phosphorylates an ion channel, causing it to open or close (see Figure 3.10C). This is the slowest of the three mechanisms, as it has the most number of steps. However, it has the longest-lasting effect and is involved in storing memories. In each mechanism a Na^+, K^+, Cl^-, or Ca^{2+} channel may be activated or inhibited, although typically this mechanism involves a Ca^{2+} or K^+ channel.

Effects on the Postsynaptic Membrane

Activation of these postsynaptic receptors, both ionotropic and metabotropic, causes changes in the permeability of ions and produces graded potentials (see Chapter 2). If the NT is linked to a Na^+ channel, Na^+ enters and depolarizes the membrane, producing an EPSP. If the NT is linked to opening a Cl^- channel, Cl^- enters and hyperpolarizes the membrane, producing an IPSP. If the NT is linked to a K^+ channel, K^+ exits the cell, also producing an IPSP. The response of each synapse is integrated with the responses of all the other synapses on the neuron, as discussed in Chapter 2.

Pharmacology of Synaptic Transmission

When considering how a drug works in the brain, it is important to realize that the drug on its own doesn't do anything novel to the neuron. Drugs bind to proteins in the neuron and either activate or inhibit their normal function. Any protein in a synapse can be a target for drug action. With this in mind, Table 3.1 shows potential targets for drug action in a neuron.

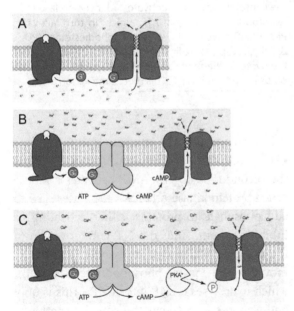

Figure 3.10 Metabotropic activation of ion channels. A. After activation by the receptor, the G-protein may directly open or close a channel. B. The G-protein may activate the production of cAMP, which may directly open or close the channel. C. cAMP may activate a protein kinase (e.g., PKA), which can phosphorylate a channel, opening or closing it.

Table 3.1 Biochemical Mechanisms of Drug Action

Drugs usually produce their effects by one of the following mechanisms:

1. Serving as a precursor for NT synthesis
2. Inhibiting NT synthesis
3. Preventing storage of the NT in vesicles
4. Stimulating the release of the NT from vesicles
5. Inhibiting fusion of vesicles at nerve terminals
6. Activating or blocking the postsynaptic receptor
7. Activating or blocking the presynaptic autoreceptors
8. Inhibiting NT degradation
9. Blocking the reuptake of the NT
10. Reversing the reuptake pump

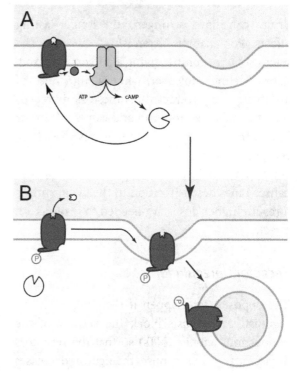

Figure 3.11 A. Activation of a receptor generally activates protein kinases in the cell. These kinases can feedback on the receptor, phosphorylating it. B. Phosphorylated receptors accumulate in pits in the membrane. These pits invaginate and withdraw these receptors from the plasma membrane to an internal pool of vesicles. Internalized receptors are no longer available to respond to NT.

Receptor Regulation

The neuron is very dynamic, always changing in response to the amount of stimulation it receives. One aspect of this is modifying the number and activity of the receptors on the postsynaptic membrane, based on the amount of NTs in the synapse.

Receptor Downregulation

When a NT activates a receptor, the activated receptor becomes a target for regulation by phosphorylation of the regulatory domain. Activation of receptors, in addition to opening ion channels, often activates intracellular kinases that phosphorylate the receptor (see Figure 3.11).

In metabotropic receptors, phosphorylation does three things. First, the phosphorylated receptor has a lower affinity for the NT, so the NT has less effect. Second, the phosphorylated receptor can no longer associate with the G-protein, also inhibiting the effect. These two processes produce desensitization. Finally, phosphorylation targets the receptor to accumulate in pits in the membrane. These pits invaginate and remove the receptors from the plasma membrane. This is *downregulation of the receptor*. If the overstimulation of the cell persists, the downregulated receptors will be degraded. This process protects the cell from becoming overstimulated.

This effect is not very pronounced under normal physiological conditions. NTs are released and taken back up quickly, and the receptors do not become overstimulated. However, drugs can have stronger and longer-lasting effects. For example, exercising can cause the release of endorphins, giving a person a relaxed, happy feeling. However, when a high dose of an opiate drug overactivates these same receptors, the effect is profound and can last for four hours. In the latter case, the neurons with these receptors will begin to withdraw them from the surface. Chronic overstimulation with opiates causes rapid desensitization to the drug, and, as a result, higher doses are needed to produce an effect.

Receptor Upregulation

The opposite can happen if the drug is an antagonist. Antagonists block the activity of the endogenous agonist (NTs) so that the receptors are less active. In response, the neuron decreases the number of receptors being withdrawn from the membrane and synthesizes more receptors. This process is called *upregulation of receptors* and leads to super sensitivity when the antagonist is removed. *Super sensitivity* means that the normal amount of NTs present now has a greater effect because there are more receptors available to interact with it.

Tolerance and Withdrawal

In the case of both agonist and antagonist drugs, the long-term result is the loss of effect of the drug due to changes in receptor numbers. This means that the dose of the drug has to be increased to produce the same effects; this is called *tachyphylaxis*. Over time, the maximal effect of the drug can no longer be reached due to the changes in receptor numbers. The change in responsiveness to the drug is called *tolerance*. This effect can be rapid and dramatic in the case of some recreational drugs (e.g., opioids).

Another consequence of a change in receptor numbers is withdrawal. When the neuron is overstimulated by an agonist, it reduces the receptors for the agonist from the membrane. When the drug is removed from the body, there are fewer receptors present on the cells to respond to the endogenous NT, so it has become less potent. The result is the opposite of the drug effect: understimulation of the cell. The opposite is true for antagonists. Chronic treatment with antagonists causes upregulation of the receptors for it. When the drug is withdrawn, the endogenous NT is now more potent (i.e., has super sensitivity) because it has more receptors to interact with. Again, the effect on the cell is the opposite of the effect of the drug. In both of these cases, the overall effect on the individual is to experience the opposite physiological effects of those produced by the drug.

This is part of the reason why chronic drug use results in withdrawal and helps explain some of the withdrawal symptoms. If a drug causes stimulation in a person, withdrawal after chronic use results in depression. This contributes to the cycle of dependence seen with drug abuse.

Summary

When an AP reaches the axon terminal, a series of events occur. The change in voltage opens VDCCs, which allow Ca^{2+} to enter. This Ca^{2+} causes vesicles containing the NT to fuse with the presynaptic membrane and release the NT. The NT fills the synapse, diffusing to the postsynaptic membrane and binding to its receptors. These receptors, whether ionotropic or metabotropic, open ion channels, producing a change in the voltage of the membrane. If the ion channels allow Na^+ in, this results in an EPSP. If the ion channels allow Cl^- in or K^+ out, the result is an IPSP. Shortly after the NT is released, it is cleared from the synapse by either being taken back up by the presynaptic membrane, by diffusing out of the synapse, or by being broken down in the synapse. Chronic stimulation or antagonism of receptor by a drug causes compensatory changes in receptor numbers, which decreases the effectiveness of the drug (tachyphylaxis).

Further Reading

Neurotransmitter release: Neher, E., and S. Takeshi. "Multiple Roles of Calcium Ions in the Regulation of Neurotransmitter Release." *Neuron* 59 (2008): 861–72.

7-TMRs: Lefkowitz, R. J. "Historical Review: A Brief History and Personal Retrospective of Seven-Transmembrane Receptors." *Trends Pharmacological Sciences* 28 (2004): 413–22.

Synaptic plasticity: Toni, N., P. A. Buchs, I. Nikonenko, C. R. Bron, and D. Muller. "LTP Promotes Formation of Multiple Spine Synapses between a Single Axon Terminal and a Dendrite." *Nature* 402 (1999): 421–5.

Glia and synapses: Araque, A., V. Parpura, R. P. Sanzgiri, and P. Haydon. "Tripartite Synapses: Glia, the Unacknowledged Partner." *Trends in Neurosciences* 22 (1999): 208–15.

Receptor regulation: Moore, C. A. C., S. K. Milano, and J. L. Benovic. "Regulation of Receptor Trafficking by GRKs and Arrestins." *Annual Review of Physiology* 69 (2007): 451–82.

Test Your Understanding

Multiple-Choice

1. When an axon bulb makes a synapse with another axon bulb, this is called
   a. axodendritic
   b. axosomatic
   c. axoaxonic
   d. all of the above

2. When an action potential reaches the axon bulb, it causes the release of neurotransmitter by
   a. activating the production of cAMP
   b. blocking the amine pump
   c. reversing the amine pump
   d. opening the VDCC

3. The role of autoreceptors is to
   a. provide feedback to inhibit neurotransmitter release
   b. bind the neurotransmitter and activate the postsynaptic membrane
   c. return the neurotransmitter to the presynaptic bulb
   d. break down the neurotransmitter in the synapse

4. The most common mechanism for removing neurotransmitter from the synapse is
   a. a presynaptic amine pump returning the neurotransmitter to the presynaptic bulb
   b. an astrocyte clearing the synapse and recycling the neurotransmitter to the presynaptic bulb
   c. enzymatically breaking down the neurotransmitter in the synapse
   d. mitochondria breaking down the neurotransmitter

5. Ionotropic receptors
    a. are also called ligand-gated ion channels
    b. respond to neurotransmitters by opening and allowing ions to pass
    c. are specific for either Na^+ or Cl^-
    d. all of the above
6. After production of cAMP, it is broken down by
    a. acetylcholinesterase
    b. phosphodiesterase
    c. G_i
    d. protein kinase A (PKA)
7. If a person is taking a high dose of a drug that blocks dopamine receptors, what is the likely response?
    a. decreased metabolism of dopamine
    b. increased metabolism of dopamine
    c. decreased numbers of dopamine receptors (downregulation)
    d. increased numbers of dopamine receptors (upregulation)
8. Desensitization is
    a. the loss of effectiveness of a drug
    b. the development of tolerance to a drug
    c. the loss of responsiveness of a cell to the neurotransmitter
    d. the upregulation of receptors for a neurotransmitter

Essay Questions

1. Describe how the presynaptic axon bulb releases neurotransmitters.
2. The venom from a marine snail is very toxic to vertebrates. In the lab, it has been shown to stop the release of neurotransmitters from all presynaptic axon bulbs, although it has no effect on the action potential in the axon. How do you think that it might work? (Hint: there are many possible answers.) Explain your answer.
3. What are three different ways that a G-protein coupled receptor could interact with an ion channel? Which pathway produces the fastest response? The slowest response?
4. What would be the effect on an axon bulb of a drug that formed a Ca^{2+} pore in the membrane, allowing Ca^{2+} to pass freely? Why would you assume this?
5. A person who smokes for the first time tends to experience much more severe effects from a cigarette than someone who smokes frequently does. Also, someone who smokes frequently experiences withdrawal symptoms that make it difficult to quit smoking. Given that the smoke contains nicotine, provide a reasonable explanation for both of these effects.

Credit

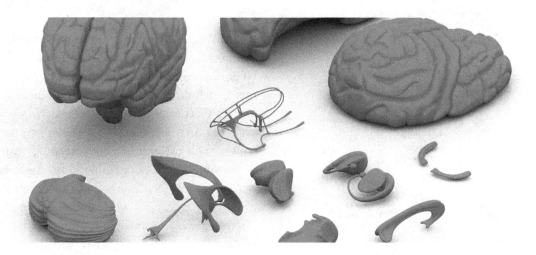

Chapter 4:
Pharmacodynamics III

Introduction

Drugs are chemicals that interact with a receptor for a specific neurotransmitter (NT) in the brain (the endogenous neurotransmitter). The drug may either mimic the NT, in which case it is an agonist for the receptor, or block it, in which case it is an antagonist. The receptors that drugs interact with are often restricted to different parts of the brain, and each part of the brain is responsible for a specific function. The effects of the drug result from which NT the drug is designed to mimic or block, where in the brain these receptors are, and the function of this part of the brain.

This chapter discusses the functions of different parts of the brain and which NTs are important in each. Learning this will make it more clear how activating or inhibiting different receptors with drugs affects the function of the brain and the experiences of the individual.

The Nervous System

The nervous system can be divided into two main parts (see Figure 4.1): the central nervous system (CNS), and the peripheral nervous system (PNS). The CNS is composed of the brain and spinal cord, while the PNS is composed of all of the nerves traveling to and from the CNS. The nerves of the PNS carry sensory information to the spinal cord, which transmits the information to the brain. The brain analyzes this sensory information and integrates it into previous experiences that are stored in the brain. It then makes decisions about how to respond to this sensory information and sends outgoing motor commands through the spinal cord to effectors (e.g., muscles, glands, etc.) in the PNS. The CNS can be further broken down into sub-regions that are each responsible for specific functions. This is the main subject of this chapter. The effects of recreational drugs are mainly created in the CNS. Side effects of recreational drugs are often created in the PNS, as some of the same NTs and receptors are used peripherally as they are in the CNS.

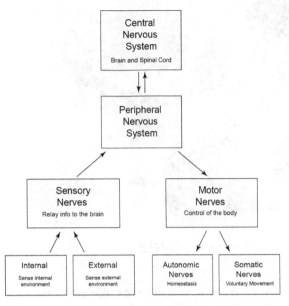

Figure 4.1 The nervous system can be divided into the central (CNS, brain and spinal cord) vs. the peripheral nervous system (PNS). The PNS includes sensory neurons that bring stimuli into the CNS from internal and external sources. The other branch of the PNS is composed of neurons that control the body (motor neurons).

There are three functional classes of neurons in the body. *Sensory neurons* are neurons that receive information from the environment. These neurons have receptors that sense the environment and initiate action potentials. This includes receptors for the classic five senses—sight, hearing, touch, taste, and smell—as well as for sensing external temperature, pain, and other stimuli. Sensory neurons also receive information from receptors monitoring the internal environment. These receptors sense the acidity of blood, oxygenation of the blood, blood pressure, body temperature, the position of limbs and the body in space, internal pain, and other important internal measures. Sensory neurons relay this information to the spinal cord.

Motor neurons relay information from the CNS to control all aspects of the body. There are two types of motor neurons: somatic and autonomic. *Somatic neurons* are responsible for voluntary control of skeletal muscles for movement, including muscle tone and balance, which are not consciously controlled. *Autonomic neurons* are responsible for the automatic control of involuntary "housekeeping" aspects of the body. They control blood pressure, heart rate, digestion, breathing, and other aspects of physiology necessary to maintain homeostasis. There are two divisions of the autonomic system: the sympathetic and parasympathetic systems. The *sympathetic system* is the "fight-or-flight" system that stimulates the body for exercise and exertion. It increases blood pressure, heart rate, and breathing and directs blood flow away from internal organs to skeletal muscles for more effective energy distribution. The *parasympathetic system* is best described as the "rest-and-digest" system. It causes slowing of the above processes for the conservation of energy when not in periods of stress or exertion.

Interneurons are the third functional class of neurons. Interneurons are found primarily in the spinal cord and brain and make up approximately 99% of the neurons in the body. These receive information from other neurons, integrate it (like computer processing), and relay the information to other interneurons or motor neurons.

The simplest kind of interneuron can be seen in a reflex arc in the spine (see Figure 4.2). Sensory information, like the heat of a flame, is brought into the spinal cord through the dorsal root (toward the back of the spine). This is passed to a spinal interneuron. If sensed, pain is minor, the interneuron passes this information up the spine to the brain to allow it to decide what to do. If the pain is intense, the information is passed up the spine but also directly to the appropriate motor neuron through the ventral root (front of the spine). This causes the contraction of muscles that pull the finger (or other limb) out of the way of the noxious stimulus. This happens instantly with no conscious input.

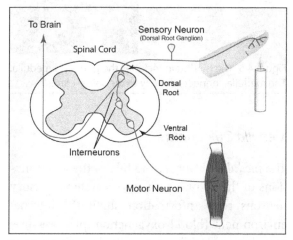

Figure 4.2 Sensory neurons bring stimuli into the spinal cord (CNS) via the dorsal root and pass it to interneurons. Interneurons decide whether to directly activate skeletal muscles or not, based on the stimulus strength, and also pass this information to ascending tracts to the brain. If skeletal muscles are engaged, the finger will be pulled back faster than the brain can respond.

Interneurons of the brain are responsible for much more complex information processing. This includes sensational awareness (conscious sensing), recognition of stimuli, memory of past events, emotional processing, and cognition. Cognition is the most complicated form of processing. Cognitive processes put the present event in the context of previous events and make rational decisions and appropriate responses. This is the highest function of the brain.

Functions of the Brain

The functions of the brain are separated into closely linked anatomical structures. The more basic functions (life support, reactive responses to stimuli) are lower down in the brain, in the brain stem on top of the spinal cord. This is made up of the medulla, pons, and the cerebellum and is sometimes called the *hindbrain* or *reptilian brain*. This is often the site of fatal drug overdose because it contains control centers for critical life functions, including respiration and cardiopulmonary control. Emotion control (fear, anger, anxiety, arousal, and euphoria/reward) is in the middle of the brain and is the function of the limbic system. This is often called the *mammalian brain*, and it is important for behavioral motivation. It is also the site of habit and addiction. Complicated cognitive functions are higher in the brain in the neocortex, often called the *primate brain*. This is the most recent evolutionarily portion of the brain and is responsible for foresight, planning, and rational control of behavior.

This separation of functions mirrors the development of the brain along our evolutionary path. Looking at Figure 4.3, you can see that more primitive brains (of fish) have relatively large portions dedicated to sensory processing (the

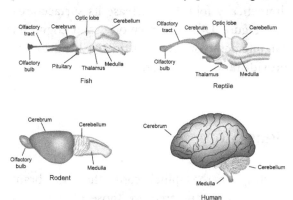

Figure 4.3 The evolutionary development of the brain in vertebrates proceeded from being designed to perform the most basic functions (autonomic regulation and reaction to the environment, medulla, thalamus and sensory reception) to the most complex functions (foresight and planning, cerebrum). Note the expansion of the cerebrum through evolution.

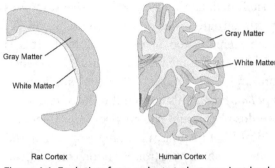

Rat Cortex   Human Cortex

Figure 4.4 Evolution from rodents to humans involved a dramatic expansion in the cerebral cortex. The cerebrum became convoluted with fissures to accommodate more surface area in the cortex within a limited brain case. Gray matter contains cell bodies of neurons while the white matter contains myelinated axons.

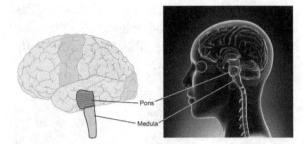

Figure 4.5 The hindbrain includes the pons and medulla. The medulla connects directly to the spinal cord.

optic lobe and olfactory bulb), life support (the medulla), and reactive and instinctive behaviors (the medulla, thalamus, and cerebellum), compared to complicated information processing (the cerebrum). Evolution through the reptilian and mammalian phases involved an expansion of the physical size of the cerebrum to cover the lower parts of the brain. This provided for more complex learned behaviors. In the human brain, the cerebrum dominates the brain and is dramatically folded to increase its surface area (see Figure 4.4). Here memories and cognition can interact to overcome instinctive behaviors to provide rational behavior.

Brain Stem

Starting at the spinal cord, the first brain structures encountered are those of the brain stem (see Figure 4.5). The *brain stem* consists of the medulla oblongata, the pons, and the cerebellum.

Medulla Oblongata

The *medulla oblongata* modulates the vital functions of the autonomic nervous system. Sensory neurons relay information about the internal environment (blood oxygenation, pH, pressure, etc.) here as well as to a higher center (the hypothalamus, discussed below). The medulla uses this information to adjust the body's physiology (heart rate, respiration, blood flow, etc.). It modulates physiological parameters to maintain homeostasis and ensure the survival of all the cells of the body. This is also the site of complex reflexes such as coughing, sneezing, swallowing, and vomiting.

The *area postrema* or *chemical trigger zone* (discussed in Chapter 1) is found in the medulla. This is a site of reduced blood-brain barrier that senses toxins in the blood and activates the vomiting reflex. Death from drug overdose is often due to either depression of the respiratory center in the medulla or stimulation of the vomit center followed by aspiration of the vomit. Thus, the medulla is central to drug overdose.

Several NTs are important in the medulla. Gamma-aminobutyric acid (GABA) and endorphins (which activate opiate receptors) are important, especially in the regulation of respiration. Drugs that affect these receptors (e.g., alcohol, barbiturates, and opiates) can cause mild depression to cessation of respiration, depending on dose.

Pons

The *pons* is a small bulbous structure located directly above the medulla. The pons is mainly white matter, which consists of tracts of myelinated axons between the body and the upper parts of the brain. As such, the main role of the pons is to coordinate movement by organizing ascending (sensory) and descending (motor) tracts. It organizes and prioritizes reflexes that maintain standing posture, balance in motion, and other physical controls, in coordination with the cerebellum.

The pons also has areas of gray matter (cell bodies organized into nuclei) that play a role in controlling breathing, facial expressions, and eye movements.

Cerebellum

The *cerebellum* is a large, bulbous structure behind the brain stem (see Figure 4.6). It coordinates with the pons and basal ganglia to smoothen movements. This is an important error-checking mechanism in balance and posture. Sensory information about the position of the body in space (proprioception) from the PNS and the vestibular system in the ear (balance) are relayed by the pons to the cerebellum. The cerebellum checks that this is correct for the motion being made and makes corrections if it is not. Learning new motor activities (e.g., riding a bike, diving into water, and playing a musical instrument) involves the cerebellum making memories of how the body should be positioned to create these movements smoothly, which are checked later when the movement is being repeated. The function of this system becomes apparent when it is

disabled by alcohol. Rapid corrections of posture are blocked, and, as a result, the individual loses balance and stumbles.

The NTs important in the cerebellum all use ionotropic receptors: GABA and glycine produce inhibitory responses, and glutamate produces excitatory responses.

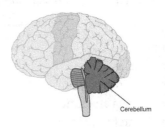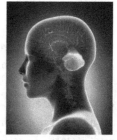

Figure 4.6 The cerebellum is a highly fissured structure with a large amount of surface area. It communicates with the pons and the midbrain to coordinate movement.

Midbrain

The *midbrain* is located between the brain stem and forebrain (see Figure 4.7). Part of the midbrain (the *tectum*) coordinates auditory and visual stimuli with movement. This area is responsible for rapid, reflexive responses to important stimuli. The other part (*tegmentum*) has two main functions. A subset of cells in this area, called the *substantia nigra*, communicate with movement centers above (*basal ganglia*) as well as the cerebellum. It then sends information down to the motor neurons to cause muscle contractions that produce voluntary movement. The substantia nigra and cerebellum help produce smooth, coordinated movements.

The tegmentum also contains cells of the ventral tegmental area (VTA). This area innervates the limbic system. The VTA is central to the motivational reward pathway that is dubbed the "pleasure circuit." Stimulation of the VTA produces euphoria and positive emotions (e.g.,

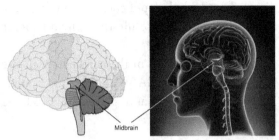

Figure 4.7 The midbrain sits on top of the pons and coordinates movement.

happiness). The function of this system will be discussed in detail in Chapter 5.

Neurons from the tegmentum release dopamine in the basal ganglia and limbic system. As a result, dopamine is vital to both movement and reward. Degradation of axon bulbs in the substantia nigra result in the movement disorder Parkinson's disease, and neurons from the VTA are intimately involved in addiction.

Another region of the midbrain is the periaqueductal gray matter (PAG). This area coordinates sensory information ascending in the brain, especially pain. It decides whether to relay this information to the cerebral cortex or not and therefore is involved in pain modulation. It also communicates with the raphe nucleus (described below) to send pain-deadening information down the spinal cord. Endorphin NTs are important here, and opioid drugs activate their receptors.

The *reticular activating system* (*RAS*) is an important area of interneurons that are spread among the pons, the medulla, and the midbrain (see Figure 4.8, in blue). Also called the *reticular formation*, these neurons regulate sleep versus wake cycles (i.e., arousal). Injury of the RAS can result in an irreversible coma. The RAS also regulates alertness, attention, and excitement. Bundles of axons from this area extend to all other areas of the brain, especially the cerebral cortex, to stimulate those areas. These are norepinephrine-releasing neurons, and stimulants such as cocaine

and amphetamines produce their effects through this neurotransmitter. Another important neurotransmitter in the RAS is acetylcholine, which is also important in arousal. The drowsiness side effect of antihistamines such as diphenhydramine (Benadryl) is produced by blocking cholinergic receptors. The RAS is particularly important in anxiety; drugs that increase its activity increase anxiety (amphetamines), and drugs that inhibit the activity decrease anxiety (benzodiazepines).

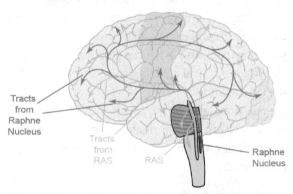

Figure 4.8 The RAS (blue) is a group of neurons that extend from the medulla through the pons to the midbrain. Axons from the RAS spread throughout the brain and produce stimulation. The raphe nucleus is similarly a group of neurons in the medulla and pons that project to most of the brain and modulate activity.

Similarly, the *raphe nucleus* is a collection of neurons whose cell bodies are found in the medulla and pons (see Figure 4.8, in red). Axons from these cells innervate many areas of the brain, including the nucleus accumbens, the dorsal striatum, and especially the cerebral cortex. These axons release the neurotransmitter serotonin and are important in regulating mood, sleep, circadian rhythms, appetite, and the thought process. Projections from the raphe nucleus also descend to the dorsal horn of the spinal cord, where they release enkephalins to modulate pain reception (more on this in Chapter 7). The effect of serotonin release in the cerebral cortex gives a person a calm, confident, positive attitude, and the raphe nucleus modulates this.

Projections from the VTA, RAS, and raphe nucleus are important modulatory factors in the brain. They release the NTs dopamine, norepinephrine, and serotonin, respectively; these NTs modulate the release of the predominant NTs in the brain, glutamate, and GABA. Many recreational drugs produce their effects by interacting with these NTs. The cell bodies of these neurons are in the brain stem–midbrain area, and their axons all pass through a central highway of ascending and descending axons called the *medial forebrain bundle*. The medial forebrain bundle allows communication from these areas to the limbic system and cerebral cortex and from these higher areas back to the midbrain.

Limbic System

The *limbic system* is a complex set of structures in the center of the brain involved in behavioral motivation and includes centers for movement, emotion, memory, and reward. Structures included in the limbic system are the thalamus, hypothalamus, basal ganglia, olfactory bulb, amygdala, hippocampus, cingulate cortex, striatum, and several other structures. Glutamate and GABA are important NTs here, as is dopamine, which modulates the latter NTs. The function of the limbic system and its role in behavioral motivation and addiction will be covered in detail in Chapter 5.

Thalamus and Hypothalamus

The *thalamus* can be thought of as the central switching area (see Figure 4.9). It is centrally located between the midbrain and the cerebrum and directs communication between them. All sensory information, except for olfactory, goes though the thalamus before being sent to the primary sensory regions in the cerebral cortex. However, rather than just passing the information to these centers, some degree of processing occurs here to determine the priority of the messages to the conscious mind. For example, if you are very focused on listening to a piece of music, you may not be aware of scenery passing as you drive down a highway, although your visual system is ensuring that you don't drive off the road. The thalamus is also important in regulating sleep-wake cycles (damage to it can result in coma) and plays a role, with the hippocampus, in memory.

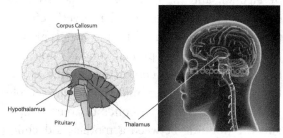

Figure 4.9 The thalamus sits in the center of the brain on top of the midbrain. The hypothalamus is directly below and in front of the thalamus. The pituitary gland is connected to the hypothalamus. The corpus callosum is composed of tracts of axons and provides communication between the right and left hemispheres of the brain.

The *hypothalamus* is a small area beneath the thalamus, as the name suggests. It is important in the regulation of physiology to maintain homeostasis and motivates simple behaviors. For example, the hypothalamus regulates blood pressure, heart rate, and gastrointestinal movements by influencing the autonomic nervous system through connections with the medulla. It regulates hunger and the feeling of being full as well as feeling thirsty. It regulates body temperature through controlling blood flow to the skin, sweating, and more complex reflexes (e.g., shivering).

The hypothalamus also regulates many hormonal functions through interactions with the pituitary gland. The hypothalamus sends "releasing factors" to the pituitary that cause it to release "stimulating" factors. These hormones, in turn, stimulate glands such as the testis and thyroid to release hormones that produce homeostatic effects in the body.

Two of the important functions that will be affected by recreational drugs are the hypothalamus's role in regulating water balance and lactation/parental attachment. Water balance is affected by antidiuretic hormone (ADH), which is released by the hypothalamus through the posterior pituitary. Release of ADH is inhibited by alcohol, and the dehydration this produces causes some of alcohol's "hangover" effects. Oxytocin is also released by the hypothalamus through the posterior pituitary and is important in regulating uterine contraction during childbirth and the letdown of milk. It also plays a role in developing emotional bonds between people and the bonding between a mother and child. MDMA (ecstasy) indirectly causes oxytocin release, producing strong emotional feelings.

Basal Ganglia

The *basal ganglia* is composed of the caudate, globus pallidus, and putamen (see Figure 4.10). These areas communicate with the substantia nigra in the midbrain to initiate and coordinate movement. Part of the basal ganglia, called the *dorsal striatum* (caudate and putamen) is important in learning behavioral patterns. This is the part of the pleasure center involved in habit formation (see Chapter 5). Another part, called the *ventral striatum*, includes the olfactory bulb and the nucleus accumbens. The *nucleus accumbens* is also part of the pleasure center and is involved in the feeling of euphoria or reward.

Acetylcholine and dopamine are important NTs in the basal ganglia.

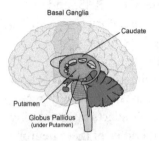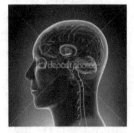

Figure 4.10 The basal ganglia sit laterally to the thalamus and are composed of the caudate, putamen, and globus pallidus (not shown, underneath the putamen).

Amygdala and Hippocampus

The *amygdala* is a major regulator of emotions (see Figure 4.11). The amygdala receives sensory information from all sources, but is directly connected to the olfactory bulb, which is why familiar smells can evoke strong emotions. Emotions such as fear, anxiety, and anger are initiated here. In response, the amygdala initiates defensive behaviors, activates the "fight-or-flight" mechanisms of the sympathetic nervous system, and stimulates the hypothalamus to release stress hormones. However, while fear conditioning is an important role of the amygdala, it is also involved in positive emotions such as happiness and sexual attraction. The amygdala is associated with memory of the events that

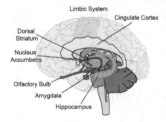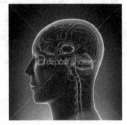

Figure 4.11 The limbic system surrounds the basal ganglia and includes the amygdala, hippocampus, nucleus accumbens, dorsal striatum, and cingulate cortex (part of the cerebral cortex).

initiated the emotions, and emotional learning in general, so that an individual remembers and learns from emotionally charged events.

The *hippocampus* lies below the amygdala and along its connections to the striatum (see Figure 4.11). It is responsible for storage of short-term memories, especially memories of events. These memories can be passed to long-term storage in the cortex or erased to make space for new memories. Anandamide (the endogenous cannabinoid) and cannabinoid receptors may be involved in this erasure. The amygdala helps in making these decisions. Unimportant memories, such as what you had for breakfast this morning, may last for a day or two, but will be gone in a year. However, what you were eating when you learned of a tragic event may be remembered for the rest of your life.

Cingulate Cortex

The *cingulate cortex* is part of the cerebrum situated inside the brain from the visible external cerebral cortex. It is a functional link between the cortex and the limbic system. The cingulate cortex can be divided into anterior and posterior portions, each having a distinct role in cognition. The cingulate wraps around the *corpus callosum*, which is a bundle of axon tracts communicating between the left and right hemispheres. It functions in directing attention to important stimuli (anterior) and tying emotions to learning and memory (posterior). Its connections to the limbic system integrate precious experiences with the feelings of reward or punishment, emotional responses to events, and memory for future repetition or avoidance. The role of the cingulate cortex will be discussed in detail in Chapter 6.

Cerebrum and Cerebral Cortex

The *cerebrum* is the largest part of the human brain and is responsible for the most advanced functions (see Figure 4.12). The cerebrum is composed of two parts (see Figure 4.4). The outer edge, or gray matter, is made up of six layers of cell bodies; this is the cerebral cortex and is where information processing occurs. Inside this gray matter is the white matter. White mater is composed of myelinated axon tracts that connect different regions of the cortex to each other and to the rest of the brain.

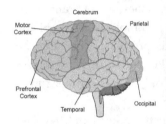 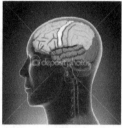

Figure 4.12 The cerebrum is the largest part of the human brain. It covers all other structures. It can be divided into 4 lobes: frontal, temporal, parietal, and occipital. The outer edge of the cerebrum is the cerebral cortex. The frontal lobe can be further divided into the motor cortex and the prefrontal cortex.

Cerebral Cortex

The *cerebral cortex* is deeply convoluted and fissured to increase its surface area and, therefore, computing power. In Figure 4.4 you can see the tremendous expansion of cortex from the rat to the human. The cortex is divided into four lobes: temporal, parietal, occipital, and frontal. The first three receive sensory input, interpret this information, and store sensory memories. The *temporal lobe* processes auditory information, the *parietal lobe* processes somatosensory information (touch, proprioception, temperature, pain, etc.), and the *occipital lobe* processes vision. The *frontal lobe* receives this information from the other lobes and uses it to decide on voluntary movement.

Each sense has a primary cortex region in its respective lobe that receives the sensory information directly from the thalamus (which has forwarded it from the ascending pathways in the brain). The primary areas produce the first conscious recognition of the sensory information. Adjacent to the primary area is the secondary or association cortex region. Cells here produce recognition of the sensory information based on pattern recognition (stored sense memories). The tertiary cortex integrates each individual sense area (from the different lobes of the brain) with the others, producing a complete picture of the experience. Part of this process is checking the new sensory information with stored memories to provide recognition of it and storage for future reference.

The frontal lobe, on the other hand, receives no direct sensory information. Information from the other three lobes is sent to the frontal lobe for conscious processing (cognition). The rearmost part of the frontal lobe contains the primary motor cortex. Neurons from this part of the brain send direct motor commands to the basal ganglia, pons, and cerebellum, which help direct voluntary movement. Adjacent secondary cortex areas store the complex instructions that pattern which muscles contract in what sequence to produce specific movements. Learning complex physical tasks, such as practicing free throws in basketball, involves making memories of these patterns and storing them here in the secondary cortex.

The *prefrontal cortex* is the site of executive function in the brain (i.e., decision making). Information from the sensory processing areas of the cortex is sent here. The prefrontal cortex checks with emotional memories in the limbic system to determine how to feel about the information. It has a store of complex memories from previous events to compare with the current situation. The prefrontal cortex then predicts future events based on the memories, emotions, and current information and decides on a course of action, relaying this to the primary motor cortex. This conscious thought produces rational behavior. It can also compare several different complex memories with the current situation to produce creative solutions to problems. This insight and planning helps produce rational rather than emotional responses to events. This is called *cognition* and will be discussed in detail in Chapter 6.

Several NTs are especially important in the cerebral cortex, and drugs that affect them are often used recreationally. Glutamate and GABA are the main excitatory and inhibitory NTs, and drugs that affect these have global effects on consciousness. Acetylcholine is an important neurotransmitter in visual perception in the primary visual cortex, as well as in both cognition and memory in the prefrontal cortex. Serotonin is released in the cortex by neurons that project from the raphe nuclei, and this input is important in controlling mood and regulating conscious thought. Norepinephrine is released here by neurons from the RAS, and it produces stimulation and excitement. Dopamine released by neurons from the VTA affects the prefrontal cortex and is important in the processing of reward. Finally, the endocannabinoid anandamide and the endogenous opioid endorphin are important NTs in the cerebral cortex, modulating thought in complex ways.

Summary

The central nervous system provides control over homeostatic maintenance of the body and voluntary control of its behavior. Many layers of control have evolved, ranging from simple reflexes and reactions to stimuli to physiological controls, to emotional control of behavior, to complex cognition to predict the future and plan for it. Imagine that you are at a party and you see a person across the room. Light reflected off the person is projected onto your retina, and sensory neurons there receive this stimulus, sending it to the thalamus. Your thalamus sees this person as important and sends this information (not information about the poster behind the person) to your primary visual cortex. The secondary cortex area deciphers the information by using stored patterns and determines that it is a person of a certain age, gender, and attractiveness. The tertiary cortex puts it together with other sensory information about this person (e.g., smell, sound of voice) to make a complete picture and sends this to the frontal lobe. The prefrontal cortex consults the limbic system to determine how you feel about this person. The limbic system compares the person to others whom you have known and decides that this person is an exciting sexual prospect and produces slight euphoria and sexual excitement to motivate you. Your limbic system prepares to mate and activates your autonomic system through the brain stem (your pupils dilate, your heart rate increases, butterflies flutter in your stomach, your genitals activate, etc.). This information is sent back to the prefrontal cortex, and it puts the brakes on. It needs more information. Is this person available? Is this person interested? Are you available? If the answers come back as yes, what is the best strategy? Is this person a good choice for a long-term relationship or just a quick mating? How does each of these prospects fit into your overall plans for the future? What are the best strategies to approach this person? However, if you are using a drug that inhibits your prefrontal cortex (e.g., alcohol), lowering your inhibitions, your prefrontal cortex may not ask these questions, and your limbic system may be in charge.

Further Reading

Vertebrate brain evolution: James L. Eilbert. "The Vertebrate Strategy for Brain Evolution." *Procedia Computer Science* 41 (2014): 233–42.

Function of cerebellum: Yu, F., Q. Jiang, X. Sun, and R. Zhang. "A New Case of Complete Primary Cerebellar Agenesis: Clinical and Imaging Findings in a Living Patient." *Brain* 138 (2014): e353. dx.doi.org/10.1093/brain/awu239.

Midbrain: Haber, S. N. "The Place of Dopamine in the Cortico-Basal Ganglia Circuit." *Neuroscience* 282 (2014): 248–57.

Amygdala: Janak, P. H., M. Kay, and K. M. Tye. "From Circuits to Behaviour in the Amygdala." *Nature* 517 (2015): 284–92.

Neurotransmitters in the cerebral cortex: Jones, E. G. "Neurotransmitters in the Cerebral Cortex." *Journal of Neurosurgery* 65 (1986): 135–53.

Brain function: Linden, D. J. *The Accidental Mind.* Cambridge, MA: Harvard University Press, 2007.

Test Your Understanding

Multiple-Choice

1. These nerves are automatic and control homeostasis in the body:
   a. peripheral nerves
   b. sensory nerves
   c. motor nerves
   d. autonomic nerves
2. These types of neurons don't receive input from other neurons:
   a. sensory neurons
   b. interneurons
   c. autonomic neurons
   d. somatic neurons
3. The highest level of function in the brain is in the
   a. reptilian brain
   b. mammalian brain
   c. primate brain
   d. none of the above
4. The chemical trigger zone, which senses toxins in the blood, is found in the
   a. medulla
   b. pons
   c. midbrain
   d. thalamus
5. Complex reflexes, such as sneezing and swallowing, are initiated by the
   a. medulla
   b. pons
   c. midbrain
   d. thalamus
6. This nucleus of cells in the midbrain sends axons to the limbic system to produce reward:
   a. RAS
   b. VTA
   c. raphe nucleus
   d. nucleus accumbens
7. This structure in the center of the brain is the functional link between the cortex and the limbic system:
   a. amygdala
   b. hypothalamus
   c. hippocampus
   d. cingulate cortex
8. This lobe of the cerebrum is responsible for visual processing:
   a. frontal lobe
   b. parietal lobe
   c. occipital
   d. temporal

Essay Questions

1. What is the role of the cerebellum? How would behavior change if a person didn't have a cerebellum?
2. What does the thalamus do?
3. The most dangerous drugs (those that produce death in overdose) are those that have effects in the brain stem. It is often difficult, if not impossible, to overdose on drugs whose effects are limited to the cerebral cortex. Why do you think this is?
4. You're a psychopharmacologist working on drugs for the central nervous system. You are studying a drug that causes lethargy in rats. What part of the brain do you think that effects? What neurotransmitter? Agonist or antagonist? Explain your answers.
5. Hallucinogens cause a disruption of normal sensory and cognitive processing. What part of the brain do they affect? What receptors may be involved?

Credits

- Fig. 4.0: Copyright © by Depositphotos / decade3d.
- Fig. 4.5b: Copyright © by Depositphotos / decade3d.
- Fig. 4.6b: Copyright © by Depositphotos / CLIPAREA.
- Fig. 4.7b: Copyright © by Depositphotos / decade3d.
- Fig. 4.9: Copyright © by Depositphotos / decade3d.
- Fig. 4.10: Copyright © by Depositphotos / decade3d.
- Fig. 4.11: Copyright © by Depositphotos / decade3d.
- Fig. 4.12: Copyright © by Depositphotos / decade3d.

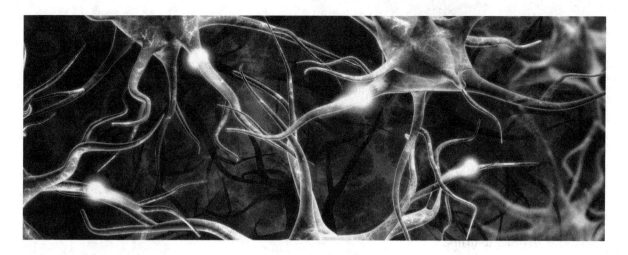

Chapter 5: Addiction

Introduction

Substance abuse first became a recognized physiological and psychological problem in the late nineteenth century. People had been addicted to substances, especially alcohol, throughout history. However, at this time medical science had advanced to the point of measuring physiological responses to stimuli. At the same time, advances in chemical separation allowed isolation of the active ingredients from plants (e.g., cocaine and morphine). This, combined with the new technology of hypodermic injection, made drugs that were previously benign into highly addictive substances. Research made it clear that these chemicals created a self-perpetuating cycle. Occasional use became chronic use, with accompanying craving and withdrawal during abstinence. This would lead to more use, higher doses, and greater craving. The addict eventually sought out the drug despite losing everything (health, wealth, family) in its pursuit. Clearly, something more than the

desire for the feeling produced by the drug was going on.

Research through the twentieth and early twenty-first centuries has been successful in identifying the neurological causes of addiction. Changes occur in the brain in response to certain drugs that make them more enticing. Some of these changes are permanent. This creates a cycle of abstinence and relapse, which intensifies the dependence on the drug. While research into the causes of addiction gives hope to finding a solution, a simple cure is elusive, and addictions still devastate many people's lives.

Abuse or Dependence?

As our understanding of addiction has evolved, so has the language used to describe it. The *Diagnostic and Statistical Manual of Mental Disorders* (*DSM*) is a document published by the American Psychiatric Association that attempts to classify all mental disorders. The first edition (*DSM–I*) was published in 1952, and it has been updated periodically to reflect the growing understanding of mental disorders. The most recent version, *DSM–V*, classifies chemical addictions as substance use disorders. This is in part to distinguish them from behavioral

Table 5.1 Alcohol Use Disorder

In the past year, have you

1. Had times when you ended up drinking more, or longer, than you intended?
2. More than once wanted to cut down or stop drinking, or tried to, but couldn't?
3. Spent a lot of time drinking? Or being sick or getting over other aftereffects?
4. Wanted a drink so badly you couldn't think of anything else?
5. Found that drinking—or being sick from drinking—often interfered with taking care of your home or family? Or caused job troubles? Or school problems?
6. Continued to drink even though it was causing trouble with your family or friends?
7. Given up or cut back on activities that were important or interesting to you, or gave you pleasure, in order to drink?
8. More than once gotten into situations while or after drinking that increased your chances of getting hurt (such as driving, swimming, using machinery, walking in a dangerous area, or having unsafe sex)?
9. Continued to drink even though it was making you feel depressed or anxious or adding to another health problem? Or after having had a memory blackout?
10. Had to drink much more than you once did to get the effect you want? Or found that your usual number of drinks had much less effect than before?
11. Found that when the effects of alcohol were wearing off, you had withdrawal symptoms, such as trouble sleeping, shakiness, restlessness, nausea, sweating, a racing heart, or a seizure? Or sensed things that were not there?

Source: Alcohol Use Disorder: A Comparison Between *DSM–IV* and *DSM–V*, http://pubs.niaaa.nih.gov/publications/dsmfactsheet/dsmfact.pdf.

addictions such as gambling, sex, and Internet gaming. This new classification replaced the *DSM–IV* separate classifications of substance abuse and substance dependence, which are both maladaptive relationships with drugs that were determined to have little clinical distinction besides severity.

Substance use disorders vary on a range from mild to severe. The distinction of severity is determined by a list of eleven criteria that are used to diagnose a substance abuse disorder. Table 5.1 shows the list for alcohol use disorder; there are other criteria specific for each substance of abuse. Mild substance use disorder is defined by exhibiting two or three of the symptoms on the list. The inclusion of more symptoms and more extreme manifestation of the symptoms warrants a more severe substance abuse diagnosis.

Neurological Source of Addictive Behavior

In 1953, postdoctoral assistants James Olds and Peter Milner, working in the lab of Donald Hebb (who will be discussed later), were experimenting with rats to determine the function of the reticular activating system (RAS) by stimulating the medial forebrain bundle. (You may remember from Chapter 4 that the RAS is involved in stimulation of the brain, helping regulate sleep-wake cycles and levels of excitement.) Because rat brains are very small structures, and not color-coded as the diagrams in Chapter 4 are, the research assistants missed their target slightly with one rat, and the electrode was placed in tracts from the VTA. After a sufficient time for healing, the rat was put into a box with the corners labeled A through D, and the electrode was attached to a stimulator that delivered shocks on the researchers' command. They found that by stimulating the electrode every time, the rat turned toward corner A, and by repeatedly stimulating it when the rat reached corner A, they could cause the rat to spend most of its time in that corner. The next day the rat automatically sought out corner A, but could be directed away from it by stimulation leading to a different corner. In a very simple and elegant way, they discovered the brain structures involved in reward-based learning.

Previous work by B. F. Skinner had developed the principle of *operant conditioning*. This is a system of reward/punishment-based learning; reward reinforces a behavior, and punishment produces aversion. He showed this through the use of a "Skinner box" (see Figure 5.1A). In this box, a reward, such as a food pellet or drink of water, is connected to an action, usually pressing a bar. Rats put into the box quickly learn to press the reward bar and remember in subsequent experiments that this is how to get a reward.

Olds and Milner modified this experiment. Instead of the bar press being linked to a food reward, it was linked to direct brain stimulation of the reward center (see Figure 5.1B). What they discovered was dramatic. Rats would press the bar rapidly, repeatedly, and to the exclusion of all other activities. Environmental cues such

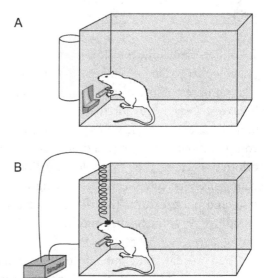

Figure 5.1 A. In the original operant conditioning experiments by B.F. Skinner, a rat is trained to push a level in order to receive the reward of a food pellet. B. In the modified Skinner experiment, an electrode is placed in the pleasure center of the rat's brain. The brain is directly stimulated by the lever press.

as food, water, grooming, and sex, which were normally rewarding experiences, were ignored because of the drive to keep hitting the bar. Rats would ignore intensely negative stimuli, such as electric shocks, in order to press the bar. The rats resembled human addicts who ignore all of the negative consequences of their actions in the drive to obtain an addictive substance. Indeed, similar results were seen when the bar press was tied to microinjections of addictive drugs such as cocaine or amphetamines. This experiment became the model to determine whether a substance was addictive or not. If a rat would self-administer the substance via bar press and return to it repeatedly, the substance was behaviorally reinforcing, which meant that it was addictive. Also, by placing the electrodes in different structures of the brain, the experiment became a way to map the circuitry involved in reward-based learning and addiction.

To understand how the limbic system works, imagine that you are a monkey living in the trees of a rainforest. Most of the food you consume is leaves. Leaves are not that nutritious. Your body can't extract much energy from them, so you spend most of the day eating to get enough calories. Because they are a low-quality food, your senses perceive leaves as having a bland taste and poor texture. This doesn't excite your emotions very much. Just another boring day, eating leaves.

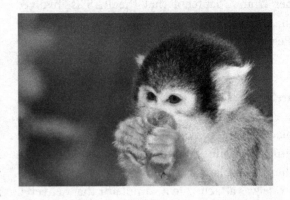

Then one day you climb out to the end of a limb and find ripe figs. Compared to leaves, these are high in easily extractable energy and protein. Your senses perceive them as tasting great. You get very happy and collect up all you can to fill your stomach. Because you just got a day's worth of calories in a half an hour, you can spend the rest of the day relaxing, building friendships, and being happy. While you are relaxing and feeling good, your brain is consolidating what you learned: trees with this shape of leaves have figs, figs are at the end of branches, ripe figs are purple (red on the inside), figs are ripe this time of year, and eating them makes you very happy. You will repeat this experience as often as possible because it makes you feel good.

On a different day, you find a bush that you have never seen before. It is loaded with red berries. Red usually means ripe and good, so you try some of the berries. They taste very bitter. You try a few more, just to make sure, and spit them out. Yuck. Shortly, you feel dizzy and sick to your stomach. Your body convulses in waves as you vomit up everything in your stomach, including the berries you swallowed. But the damage is done. Some of the berries got into your system and now you feel really bad. You find a quiet place to rest while they wear off, and your brain consolidates this memory: not all red things are good, this particular bush is really bad, and bitter taste means spit out—don't swallow. You will avoid this bush and feel fear when you see another like it.

The Limbic System

The limbic system includes several structures in the center of the brain (briefly discussed in Chapter 4). It functions to produce feelings and emotions in a person in response to external stimuli. It also records the events responsible for the emotions (environmental cues), which allows the person to learn from the events, and passes important memories to long-term storage. This produces motivational reward. It was evolutionarily designed to direct a person's behavior toward actions that support the goals of evolution: survival and reproduction. Thus, events that are evolutionarily good (e.g., eating, drinking, sex, childcare, and social promotion) are rewarded with good, positive feelings (joy, relaxation, and happiness). Events that are evolutionarily bad (e.g., encountering dangerous animals, falling from high places, losing a loved one, or social demotion) are punished with negative feelings (fear, anger, or sadness). This "carrot-and-stick" approach of the limbic system directs a person toward achieving important life goals.

The learning aspect of the system is what makes animals adaptive to their environment. It would be impossible for evolution to code responses to all of the specific events that are necessary for survival and reproduction in every possible environment. Thus, by both rewarding good behavior and making memories of the environmental cues leading to it, the limbic system makes behavior adaptable. In addition, environmental cues produce a reward even before the behavior is performed to lead the individual to seek that reward. This is "craving" and is an important part of the addictive process.

Addictive drugs more or less highjack this mechanism. These drugs, in one way or another, directly stimulate positive feelings and emotions through the limbic system. Rather than rewards coming from events such as doing well in school, falling in love, or having a great meal, a much more intense reward comes from doing the drug. Environmental cues such as the time of day, friends in abuse, drug paraphernalia, or use of other drugs associated with the addiction (e.g., coffee and cigarettes) activate cravings that lead to drug use. This maladaptive behavior becomes the sole focus of a person's life, to the exclusion of socially acceptable behaviors, and in spite of very negative consequences (losing a job, breaking up a marriage, or abandonment of a child). People resort to behaviors that would have previously been repellant, such as armed robbery or prostitution, in order to maintain the drug habit. Recovery becomes difficult due to withdrawal symptoms and permanent changes in the brain. Sustained abstinence is difficult due to hardwired cravings for the drug.

Structures of the Limbic System

There are several brain structures that are especially important in the limbic system. It starts in the ventral tegmental area (VTA) in the midbrain, which is the central control of the system. Neurons with cell bodies here project axons to stimulate five important areas: the nucleus accumbens (NA), amygdala, dorsal striatum (DS), hippocampus, and prefrontal cortex (PFC; see Figure 5.3). Stimuli that increase excitability in the cell bodies of the VTA (i.e., produce EPSPs) cause action potentials in their axons, which release the neurotransmitter dopamine in these five areas. Stimuli that decrease excitability in these neurons (i.e., produce IPSPs) decrease the rate of action potential firing and inhibit the release of dopamine.

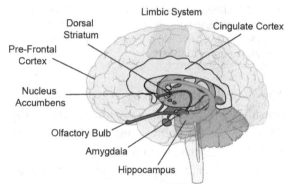

Figure 5.3 This is a representation of the structures of the limbic system (reproduced from Chapter 4).

Each structure in the limbic system plays a role in the process of behavioral adaptation (see Figure 5.4). The NA is the main reward center. It produces the feeling of euphoria or joy. The amygdala produces emotions (fear, anger, sadness, sexual excitement, and happiness) and coordinates emotional responses of the body. The hippocampus is the site of short-term storage of memories, especially memories of events. If these events are emotionally significant (either good or bad), they later will be moved to long-term storage in the cerebral cortex.

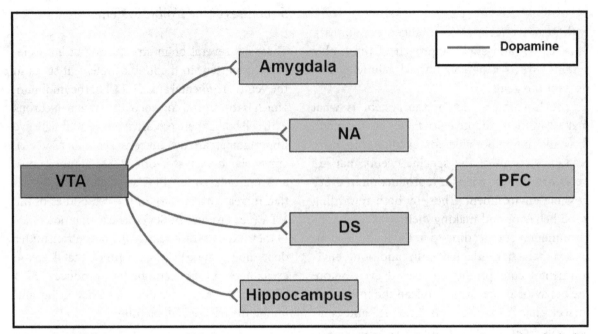

Figure 5.4 Limbic System Function. This is a schematic representation of the functional connections within the limbic system. Dopamine-releasing neurons project from the VTA to the five areas of the pleasure circuit. The NA feeds back on the VTA with GABA releasing neurons. Other areas of the circuit (amygdala, DS, hippocampus, and PFC) project glutamate-releasing neurons to the NA.

Alternatively, they will be erased if they are considered to be emotionally unimportant. The DS is the site of habit formation (i.e., learned behaviors that lead to events). Finally, the PFC is the site of learning, planning, and integration of events. The PFC puts events into context with memories and prioritizes which events are most important. This prioritizing is based on determining the salience (importance) of the event. Excitation in the VTA causes the release of dopamine in all five of these areas.

Any biological mechanism that produces a response has a feedback mechanism to prevent the response from going out of control. There are complicated networks of feedback pathways in the limbic system that inhibit overstimulation (see Figure 5.5). In one, cell bodies in the NA that are simulated by the neurons from VTA, project axons back to the VTA to release the inhibitory NT GABA when stimulated. This is negative feedback; it decreases action potentials in the VTA and therefore decreases VTA stimulation of dopamine release in the NA. Other areas of the limbic system (the amygdala, PFC, DS, and hippocampus) project excitatory axons (glutamate) to these GABAergic neurons in the NA, stimulating their inhibitory effect on the VTA. There are also neurons in the PFC that project glutamate-releasing axons to the VTA, stimulating the VTA to produce reward. This is positive feedback; these glutamate-releasing neurons anticipate rewarding events. They are very important in the craving that accompanies addiction. In addition, there are excitatory pathways from the DS to the NA that stimulate reward. The DS is responsible for reinforcing behaviors (habits) that lead to reward. This pathway produces reward to encourage behavior before they are performed and is important in the compulsiveness of drug-seeking behaviors.

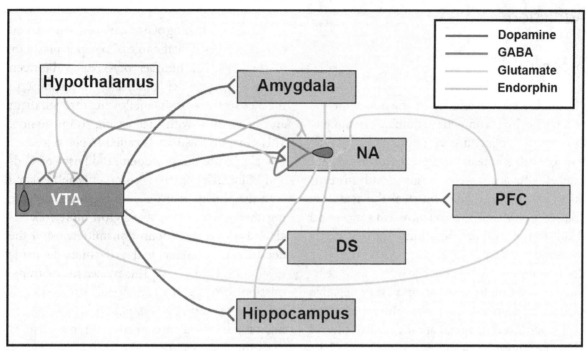

Figure 5.5 Feedback Pathways of the Limbic System. The NA feeds back on the VTA with inhibitory GABA releasing neurons. Other areas of the circuit (amygdala, DS, hippocampus, and PFC) project stimulatory glutamate-releasing neurons to these GABA neurons in the NA. The PFC also projects glutamate-releasing axons to stimulate the VTA. The hypothalamus projects inhibitory endorphin-releasing axons to the GABA neurons in the VTA and NA to inhibit GABA release. This increases dopamine release.

Finally, endorphin-releasing neurons project from the hypothalamus and make axoaxonic connections with GABA-releasing neurons in both the VTA and NA. Endorphins here activate μ-opioid receptors that inhibit the release of GABA. By inhibiting the inhibitory neurotransmitter GABA, endorphins cause an increase in the dopamine released, both directly in the NA and throughout the limbic system through the VTA. This disinhibition of dopamine release produces reward and is central to the addictive qualities of opiate drugs (see Chapter 8).

Biological Set Point of Mood

While the limbic system is called the reward center, it is important to realize that it does more than just "light up" when a positive event is experienced. The limbic system, and especially the amygdala, sets the overall mood of a person. Just as the body has a set point for core temperature (37°C or 98.6°F), it also has a set point for feeling emotionally normal. You have up days and down days, relative to a basal set point. This set point is based on tonic, basal release of neurotransmitters in the limbic system and can be changed. Drug addiction resets the average set point lower (i.e., depression and anxiety) in the absence of the drug. This withdrawal is one of the triggers of drug seeking and will be discussed below.

Addiction

Drug Craving

The limbic system and its interaction with the cortex prioritizes competing stimuli. For example, looking down a menu at a restaurant, a salad may look good, but a steak looks great. Previous experiences with steaks were awesome, and this produces a strong craving for the steak the next time you see it on the menu. You have had some good salads in the past, but the stimulus produced by the steak creates a stronger craving than the salad does. Every positive experience with a food reinforces the desire to repeat it, and every negative experience decreases the desire. The descriptions of the items on the menu are the environmental cues that stimulate the limbic system (through its connections with the cortex, which is mediating these stimuli) to activate craving for the items. Looking down a menu is like testing out which cravings are strongest on any particular night. The cortico-limbic connection creates craving by producing a slight reward before the event takes place. This leads you to the choice that you make, just as Olds and Milner directed their rat to a specific corner by stimulating it when it turned in that direction.

Intense craving is part of what makes a drug addictive. If the drug produces a wonderful feeling but there is no craving in its absence, a person could do the drug recreationally without eventually doing it to the exclusion of all else. But intense euphoria strengthens the craving pathways. The more intense the rush of the drug (i.e., the rapid onset and high peak of euphoria), the greater the neuroadaptation to repeat the experience. The other part of addiction is compulsive drug seeking; this is a drive to get the thing that will satisfy the craving, and it is strengthened to the point where it is impossible to resist.

The strengthening of particular environmental cues is explained by the role of synaptic plasticity in learning. The number of synapses between neurons is dynamic; it increases in response to the increased transmission flowing through them and decreases with decreasing transmission. This synaptic plasticity is called *Hebb's rule*, after Donald Hebb, the postdoctoral adviser of Olds and Milner. Hebb's rule is commonly abbreviated with the phrase "neurons that fire together, wire together." Hyperactive axons grow more collaterals and release more neurotransmitters, while the dendrites they interact with grow more dendritic spines (see Figure 5.6). This makes future transmission through this connection stronger. This process is called *neuroadaptation*, the remodeling of the neural architecture in response to the stimuli. It is a form of learning that can be permanent.

The Cortex and the Salience Network

The *cortex* is the decision-making part of the brain. It receives all of the sensory information available, both external cues and internal states, and relates this to past experiences (long-term memory) and potential future consequences. Myriad interconnections between different parts of the cortex prioritize actions based on the salience (importance) to the person, now and in the future. This function is performed by a network of interacting brain regions of the cortex called the salience network (SN), which will be discussed more in Chapter 6.

The cortex has both activating and inhibiting pathways. The activating pathways make the person crave or desire something, increasing its emotional importance. The inhibiting pathways put on the brakes. They help dampen immediate emotional desires if it is determined that long-term rewards will be greater than the immediate

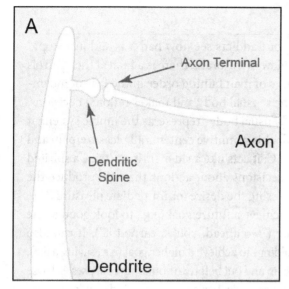

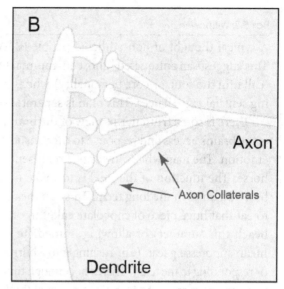

Figure 5.5 A. An axon terminal of one neuron synapses with a dendritic spine of another. B. Increased transmission through the synapse causes the outgrowth of axon collaterals and more dendritic spines. This results in more synapses and a greater connection between the neurons. This is a type of memory formation.

pleasure. This is called *willpower*—the ability to override wants and desires to accomplish a more important goal. (This long-term decision-making control is discussed more in Box 5.2.)

Addictive drugs build strong neural pathways. These drugs are so effective at increasing dopamine in the limbic system that the cortex sees this extremely pleasurable event as more important than other stimuli. This supranormal stimulus reinforces activating pathways through synaptic plasticity. When the cortex experiences environmental stimuli (cues) that previously led to the reward, it stimulates the VTA through glutamate-releasing axons. This causes pleasure (even in the absence of the drug) and the desire for more. The craving that is felt is caused by stimulation through the cortex-VTA connection. It "primes" the limbic system to receive more stimulus. This creates the impulsive drug-seeking behavior. Active drug-seeking pathways override the inhibitory PFC pathways that should keep excessive behavior in check. (The part of the cortex involved is the insula, which

will be discussed in Chapter 6 as part of the salience network.)

The Dorsal Striatum

At the same time, strengthened connections between the NA and DS create compulsive drug-seeking behavior. The DS is the center of habit formation, and strengthening its connection to the NA converts the motivation for drug seeking from a reward-based activity to a habit-based activity. The addict automatically seeks the drug, irrespective of reward. Just as a person with obsessive-compulsive disorder may be incapable of stopping hand washing (which produces a reward in his or her experience), the drug-addicted person becomes incapable of inhibiting behaviors leading to drug use. This type of compulsive activity is one of the criteria mentioned above for the diagnosis of substance use disorder. Like the PFC, the DS creates the sense of reward in the NA before the drug is actually taken. This is another "priming" reward

Box 5.2: Willpower

A typical thought of non-addicted people is "Why don't addicts see how bad it is and just stop?" This suggests an antiquated "ghost-in-the-machine" view of the brain; there is a man at the controls (call him the soul, or core personality) who is in charge of maintaining order in the face of incoming sensual experiences. This man is separate from the sensual body and makes rational decisions.

There is some truth in this view of the brain. The "sensual body" represents the limbic system; it is the brain's access and response to the sensual world. This primitive center is all pleasure/pain and emotion. The man who is in control represents the PFC; it acts like a rider sitting astride a spirited horse. The function of the PFC is to make rational decisions about actions that will produce the best outcomes in the long term. This can mean suppressing the desire for immediate pleasure (e.g., to eat that huge piece of chocolate cake) in order to achieve a future goal (e.g., to look good at the beach this summer) or allowing immediate pleasure ("Go ahead, you've earned it"). It can also mean suppressing fear[1] (e.g., rushing into a burning building) to achieve a higher goal (e.g., saving a life), or responding to the fear ("There's not enough time to get in and out before the building collapses"). These two systems correspond to rapid, emotional thinking and slow, deliberate thinking. Both are important, but on balance it is better to have the deliberate thinker in control.

However, these two systems are not separate. Just as the PFC can exert control over the limbic system (top-down control), the limbic system can overwhelm the PFC (bottom-up control). In addiction, neuroplasticity has changed the relationship between these two systems. PFC pathways have been weakened, and limbic pathways have been strengthened. In particular, chronic drug use weakens the ventromedial PFC (the part of the brain right behind your eyes). It integrates past experiences with current stimuli to predict future events. The addicts with the worst long-term ability to get and stay clean are deficient in this region; fMRI studies show that they have defects in their ventromedial PFC. There is a significant reduction in gray matter here, and the result is that addicts lack the ability to delay gratification. This is called "myopia of the future." They will always choose immediate pleasure, despite the promise of greater future reward or future pain. Functional studies show that they make similar responses to choices as do people who have had strokes or other damage to this area. They lack this important area for cognitive control.

The ventromedial PFC may be analogous to the arms of a man riding a horse. Addiction weakens the man's arms, so he can no longer control the reigns; the horse of his limbic system runs free, driven by the cravings of the PFC and compulsion of the dorsal striatum. The problem isn't that the man in charge is weak-willed; it's that he lost his ability to exert his will. That part of the brain is not functioning. Hoping that addicts will simply straighten out when they see the consequences of their actions doesn't work. The drugs have weakened the specific brain center that performs this control function.

---

[1] "Bran thought about it. 'Can a man still be brave if he's afraid?' 'That is the only time a man can be brave,' his father told him." From *A Song of Fire and Ice*, by George R. R. Martin.

that can be greater than the reward produced by the drug itself.

Anhedonia

Changes in the PFC also decrease the craving for and pleasure produced by normal stimuli, making everyday pleasures meaningless. The limbic system becomes rewired to desire only the supranormal stimulus of the drug and to deprioritize normal stimuli. This produces *anhedonia*, or the lack of joy from normal life, in the absence of the drug. This can last weeks to months after withdrawal from the drug is over and is one of the factors involved in relapse. Anhedonia is also related to a depletion of dopamine and decrease in dopamine receptors in the limbic system (discussed below), although it lasts long after these factors have recovered.

Withdrawal

Another aspect of addiction is the desire to avoid withdrawal. *Withdrawal syndrome* is a set of physical and emotional feelings in the absence of the drug. Part of the withdrawal is due to the downregulation of the reward pathway. Overstimulated dopamine receptors are retrieved from the dendrite membrane (see Figure 3.11). If the drug causes an increase in the neurotransmitter release, then another aspect of the downregulation is depletion of the axon bulbs of neurotransmitter. Together these mechanisms result in less pleasure being produced by the same dose of the drug. Higher doses must be taken to produce euphoria, and the effect is not as pleasurable (tachyphylaxis). In addition, maintaining a normal, basal level of emotion is difficult in the absence of the drug.

The natural pathways are no longer capable of making the person feel normal, and depression follows.

The Anti-Reward System

Another part of withdrawal is the activation of a parallel pathway to the reward circuit, the anti-reward circuit, which acts to diminish reward. This is the basis of the opponent process theory of addiction (see Figure 5.7). Normally the anti-reward pathway is another feedback mechanism to stop hedonistic tendencies from overcoming rational control. The predominant feeling associated with the anti-reward circuit is *dysphoria*, which is a feeling of unease, dissatisfaction, or depression.

The anti-reward circuit begins in the amygdala, which extends axons to the thalamus/hypothalamus, NA, and RAS. The neurotransmitters involved are dynorphin, corticotropin-releasing factor (CRF), and norepinephrine. Dynorphin is an endogenous opiate that activates κ-opiate receptors in the NA, producing dysphoria. CRF is a peptide hormone that activates the pituitary to release adrenocorticotropic hormone (ACTH), which in turn causes the release of cortisol from the adrenal glands. Cortisol is the major stress hormone in the body; whenever you are stressed, cortisol levels elevate. Cortisol decreases the PFC functioning (rational thought) that normally exerts control over the pleasure-seeking pathways. This is one reason why stress is one of the triggers for relapse (see below). CRF is also used in the CNS as a neurotransmitter. Axons from the amygdala project to the RAS and stimulate it by releasing CRF. This is part of the stress response and results in the release of norepinephrine by the RAS, stimulating the entire brain. (The CRF-stress pathways will be discussed further in Chapter 8.)

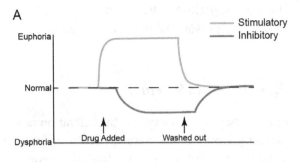

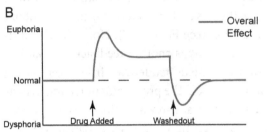

Figure 5.7 A. Addictive drugs produce euphoria by activating the reward pathway. Compensations anti-reward mechanisms are then activated, delayed behind the euphoric response. After washout of the drug, the reward Opponent Process Theory of Addiction. A. Addictive drugs produce euphoria by activating the reward pathway. Compensatory anti-reward mechanisms are then activated, delayed behind the euphoric response. After washout of the drug, activation of the reward pathway stops while activation of the anti-reward pathways continues for a period of time. B. The overall effect on mood is the difference between the reward and anti-reward pathways. The lasting anti-reward effects produce depression after the drug has been removed.

The reward and anti-reward pathways oppose each other and are regulated in opposition. When the reward pathway is activated to produce happiness, the anti-reward is activated to bring the individual down again. The reverse is also true. When the anti-reward pathway is activated (through fear, sadness, or anxiety), the reward pathway is also activated. This is why sad or scary movies and amusement park rides are enjoyable. They produce intense negative emotions that are followed by pleasurable withdrawal.

Both of these pathways respond to overstimulation by addictive drugs, but in opposite

directions (see Figure 5.8). The reward pathway becomes downregulated, as discussed above. On the other hand, the anti-reward system is augmented. Normally this system produces a low feeling when the drug wears off. In the addict, the lows are much lower. Neuroadaptation increases the amount of transmission in the anti-reward system that results in profound depression in the absence of the drug.

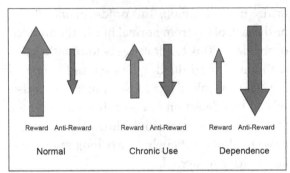

Figure 5.8 Under normal conditions, activation of the reward pathway also causes activation of the anti-reward pathway, which originate in the amygdala.

Over time the changes in these two systems produce a new emotional set point (see Figure 5.9). An occasional user will experience the high of the drug, then the low of withdrawal, followed by a return to normal in a short period of time. The chronic user will experience a lower high, then depression, followed by extended dysphoria. The chronic user needs to take the drug to get back to normal functioning. This is called *dependence*; the user needs to take the drug just to break even. As dependence takes over, the addict compulsively seeks the drug to avoid pain rather than to feel pleasure.

The dysphoria created by the lowered emotional set point can last months to years after complete abstinence from the drug. It is another source of anhedonia and another factor in relapse.

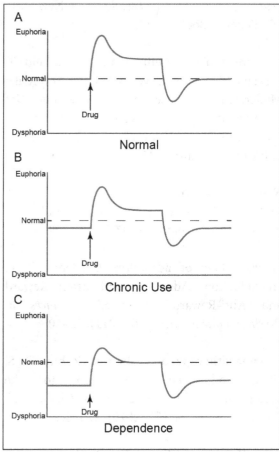

Figure 5.9 An Emotional Set Point. A. The reward and anti-reward pathways set the overall emotional mood of a person, which can be considered to be a set point. Drugs dramatically elevate mood, which activates compensatory anti-reward mechanisms. The compensatory mechanisms temper the euphoria and cause a depression, or withdrawal, after the drug wears off although the person eventually returns to a "normal" baseline. B. Chronic drug use weakens the reward pathways and strengthens the anti-reward pathways, resulting in lower highs and lows. Overall, baseline becomes lower than normal. C. Long-term, chronic use creates a new, lower emotional set point. The addict depends on the drug to regain a "normal" state and descends into depression in the absence of the drug.

Relapse

The multiple neuroadaptations produced by chronic overstimulation of the reward pathway causes relapse to be a recurrent phenomenon in recovery. One re-exposure to the drug after being clean stimulates the NA, reactivates the craving pathways from the PFC, and compulsion from the DS. The cycle of addiction starts all over again. Even exposure to another drug can reactivate these pathways and restart the original addiction. Relapse after abstinence greatly enhances the craving, making the addiction worse this time. Thus a small "taste" of the drug during abstinence typically results in full-blown addiction again, which is more intense and harder to stop. Each cycle of rehabilitation and relapse strengthens the grip of the addiction.

Another stimulus that causes craving and relapse is exposure to the environmental cues that are remembered to precede the drug use. This includes physical surroundings (e.g., being back in the old neighborhood), former friends in the abuse, activities associated with drug use, paraphernalia associated with drug use (pipes, needles, etc.), and other drugs that were taken at the same time. This activates the "priming" stimuli to the VTA and weakens the resolve to avoid the drug.

Finally, stress is also a predictor of relapse. Stress-induced relapse is due to activation of the amygdala-CFR-RAS-NE pathway discussed above as part of the anti-reward circuit. Stress, through CRF, weakens PFC control. Drugs relieve the stress by activating the pathways previously found to produce pleasure.

Summary

The pleasure circuit of the limbic system is important to the adaptability of an animal. It helps guide behavior to activities that support the animal's survival and reproduction. Addictive drugs highjack this mechanism and realign its purpose to highly maladaptive drug-seeking behaviors. Addictive drugs all have the ability to hyperstimulate the pleasure circuit, either indirectly by stimulating the VTA or directly by increasing dopamine in the VTA's synapses with the NA (euphoria), DS (habit), amygdala (mood), hippocampus (memory), and PFC (foresight and planning). This produces a feeling of euphoria and happiness. Compensatory feedback mechanisms follow in the absence of the drug, leading to depression in withdrawal. Chronic overstimulation of the pleasure center causes neuroadaptation to the supranormal stimulus. This includes a lowering of the mood set point (depression), decreasing the pleasure derived from normal stimuli (anhedonia), obsessive focus on drug seeking (craving), and habitual return to the drug (compulsiveness). Neuroadaptation is permanent and makes relapse common, even after a prolonged period of abstinence. Re-exposure to the drug (or other euphoria-inducing drugs), to the environment where the drugs were taken, or to stress causes a rebound of the craving and compulsive behavior, and reinforces these pathways. The addict is then in a worse place than he or she was before becoming abstinent.

Further Reading

DSM-V: American Psychiatric Association. *Diagnostic and Statistical Manual of Mental Disorders.* 5th ed. Arlington, VA: American Psychiatric Publishing, 2013.

The pleasure circuit: Linden, D. *The Compass of Pleasure: How Our Brains Make Fatty Foods, Orgasm, Exercise, Marijuana, Generosity, Vodka,* *Learning, and Gambling Feel So Good.* New York, NY: Penguin Books, 2011.

The amygdala: Cunningham, W. A., and T. Kirkland. "The Joyful, yet Balanced, Amygdala: Moderated Responses to Positive but Not Negative Stimuli in Trait Happiness." *Social and Cognitive Affective Neuroscience* 9 (2013): 760–6. doi: 10.1093/scan/nst045.

Neuroadaptation: Koob, G. F., and N. D. Volkow. "Neurocircuitry of Addiction." *Neuropsychopharmacology* 35 (2010): 217–38.

Neurobiology of addiction: Gardener, E. L. "Introduction: Addiction and Brain Reward and Anti-Reward Pathways." *Advances in Psychosomatic Medicine* 30 (2011): 22–60.

Pharmacotherapy of addiction: Zahm, D. S. "Pharmacotherapeutic Approach to the Treatment of Addiction: Persistent Challenges." *Molecular Medicine* 107 (2010): 276–80.

Addiction: Wiers. R. W., and A. W. Stacy, eds. *Handbook of Implicit Cognition and Addiction.* Thousand Oaks, CA: Sage Publications, 2006.

Test Your Understanding

Multiple-Choice

1. What is the biological role of the limbic system?
    a. to produce pleasure
    b. to produce behavioral adaptation
    c. to respond to drugs
    d. to generate emotions

2. Stimulation of the limbic system is initiated in the
   a. VTA
   b. nucleus accumbens
   c. dorsal striatum
   d. hippocampus
3. The part of the limbic system associated with memory of events is the
   a. amygdala
   b. VTA
   c. nucleus accumbens
   d. hippocampus
4. The part of the limbic system mainly associated with euphoria and addiction is the
   a. amygdala
   b. VTA
   c. hippocampus
   d. nucleus accumbens
5. The neurotransmitter associated with feedback inhibition in the limbic system is
   a. endorphin
   b. dopamine
   c. glutamate
   d. GABA
6. The part of the brain that produces cravings is the
   a. prefrontal cortex
   b. dorsal striatum
   c. nucleus accumbens
   d. VTA
7. Synaptic plasticity involves
   a. neurons growing more dendritic spines
   b. axons growing more collaterals
   c. permanent changes in neural pathways
   d. all of the above
8. In addiction, the dorsal stratum is responsible for
   a. lowering the set point of mood
   b. constant cravings
   c. compulsive drug use
   d. all of the above

Essay Questions

1. What is the difference between the experiments of Skinner and Olds and Milner? Why were the latter's experiments important in addiction research?
2. Name the structural parts of the limbic system and the function of each. How do these functions relate to the role of the limbic system?
3. A research lab has developed a drug that is an antagonist at dopamine receptors. What do you think that effect of this drug on the brain would be? What side effects is it likely to produce?
4. Reward deficiency syndrome (RDS) is a newly designated condition for people who are genetically predisposed to having low levels of dopamine-related reward in the brain. Some say that this syndrome may underlie addictions. Why do you think this may be?
5. What is meant by the "emotional set point of mood"? How does this enter into the process of addiction?

Credits

- Fig. 5.0: Copyright © by Depositphotos / 100502500.
- Fig. 5.2: Copyright © by Depositphotos / mamopictures.

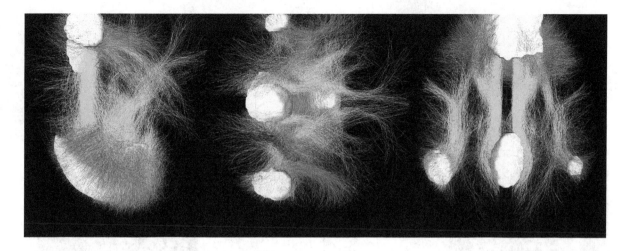

Chapter 6: Cognition

Introduction

What is cognition? What exactly is that voice in our heads? Where does it come from? How does it help us understand the world, see ourselves as distinct from the world, and predict the future? How does our thinking go wrong in disease states? And how is it affected by drugs?

These are some of the most exciting questions being asked today in the field of neuroscience. Some studies are developing an understanding of how axons crisscross the cortex, connecting different regions that each have a specific function. Other studies show which of these regions of the brain "light up" when specific tasks are being performed. Connections between these active areas produce distinct functional networks that are specific for different tasks and modes of thinking. These separate networks send information to each other. In the rapid trading of information between different areas, we respond to the environment, respond to our feelings, reflect on the

past, predict the future, and decide on our actions. In the course of this, our personality emerges. Blocking or enhancing these connections with drugs produces altered modes of thinking.

In the currently accepted model, there are three main networks involved in second-to-second processing (see Figure 6.1). The *task-positive network* (*TPN*) is directed toward receiving external stimuli, coordinating this with information in working memory, and performing a goal-directed task. This is used for focused attention tasks, such as taking an exam or playing a game. The *default-mode network* (*DMN*) is active when a person is relaxed and ruminating. This mind-wandering state is self-reflective and orients you with your world (past, present, and future). In the middle of these (both functionally and anatomical) is the *salience network* (*SN*). The SN receives sensory information about the world and your emotional state and decides what is most important for you to do now. It is the control center that directs your thinking toward either the TPN or DMN. The neurons in these networks, which reside in the associative cortex of their respective regions of the cerebral cortex (gray matter), are connected by myelinated axons (white matter). In the process of passing information around, these networks produce your personality and conscious thought.

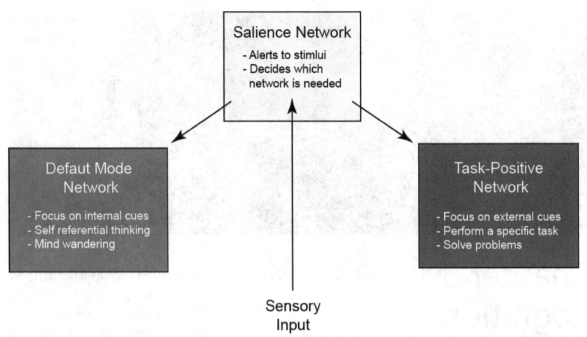

Figure 6.1 This is a general overview of how cognition is controlled by the cerebral cortex. Sensory input, internal and external somatosensory as well as emotional sensing (limbic), enters conscious awareness in the Salience Network. This determines which mode of thinking is needed. Default Mode Network is a relaxed, mind-wandering, self-reverential mode of thinking. Task Positive Network is a focused, external mode that is directed toward performing a task.

Methods of Measuring Brain Activity

Before discussing the networks of the brain and modes of thinking, it is important to understand how studies are done to learn about these processes. This will help you appreciate where this knowledge came from and critically assess the limitations of the science.

Electroencephalography (EEG) and magneto-encephalography (MEG) are methods of measuring electrical activity in the cortex. Positron emission tomography (PET) and functional magnetic resonance imaging (fMRI) are methods of creating three-dimensional images of the activity in the brain. Diffusion tensor imaging (DTI) is an MRI imaging process used to produce accurate representations of the axonal connections in the brain.

For *EEG* recordings, electrodes are placed on the scalp (see Figure 6.2). These electrodes can detect electrical activity on the surface of the cortex and down into the sulci (folds of the cortex). The advantage of this method is that it gives an instantaneous reading of brain activity (in the order of milliseconds). This makes it easy to relate what the person is experiencing to contemporaneous brain activity. It is also a very inexpensive method of recording brain activity. The major limitation is that it has very poor spatial resolution (i.e., geographic isolation); many, many neurons contribute to the recordings, and pinpointing exact areas of activation is not possible. Also, EEG can measure only from the surface of the cortex; it cannot detect activity in the underlying layers.

MEG similarly measures activity in the surface of the cortex on a very short time scale (<1 millisecond). The measurements are based on magnetic fields created by the electrical activity in neurons. MEG has greater special resolution

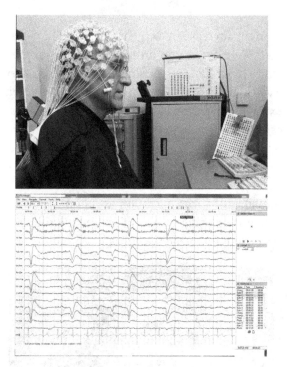

Figure 6.2 The electroencephalogram (EEG) is a measure of the electric activity on the surface of the brain. It allows for very good temporal resolution of signals, but relatively poor geographic isolation of the signal.

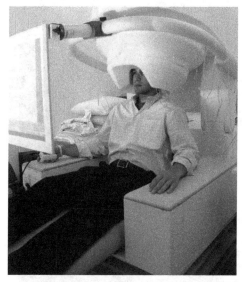

Figure 6.3 Magnetoencephalography (MEG) measures electrical brain activity based on the magnetic fields that it produces. This provides good temporal and geographic resolution, but is unable to penetrate beyond the outer layers of the cortex.

than EEG across the surface of the cortex (in the range of centimeters), but is unable to penetrate beyond the surface. MEG also requires much more complicated and expensive equipment, as well as extensive shielding to eliminate magnetic fields produced by the electrical equipment in the lab (see Figure 6.3).

PET and fMRI are three-dimensional imaging techniques. They are often based on changes in the amount of metabolic activity in different regions of the brain while the subject is performing tasks or at rest. Neuronal activity is very energy intensive. While the brain represents only 5% of the body mass, it uses 20% of the body's total energy output. When brain activity in an area increases, it requires more glucose and oxygen. PET and fMRI measure these changes.

PET is capable of measuring activity in all areas of the brain in three dimensions at millimeter resolution (see Figure 6.4). It is based on measuring the radioactive emissions of a tracer chemical that is injected immediately before recording. Often, the tracer is an analog of a chemical naturally used in metabolism. For example, [F^{18}] fludeoxyglucose can be used to measure energy usage. It is glucose with one OH group replaced by radioactive fluorine. More metabolically active cells will take up more glucose and [F^{18}] fludeoxyglucose with it. The PET scanner measures the concentration of [F^{18}] fludeoxyglucose in different regions by detecting the radioactivity given off. A computer analyzes these emissions and generates a three-dimensional model of metabolic hotspots in the brain. [O^{15}] H$_2$O can also be used in PET. This is water that contains a radioactive isotope of oxygen; it can be used to detect changes in blood flow (similar to fMRI, described below).

The main limitation of PET studies is time resolution. Activity is measured in the order of tens of seconds to minutes. This seriously limits

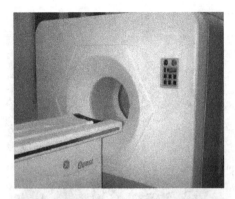

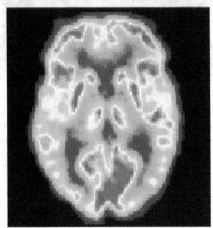

Figure 6.4 Positron Emission Tomography (PET) measures radioactive emission from a tracer chemical injected prior to recording. It provides excellent three dimensional geographical isolation of a signal, but slow temporal resolution.

than the increase in oxygen consumption. So, as metabolic activity in an area increases, oxygen content paradoxically increases as well. Another way to look at this is that the amount of oxygen extracted from the blood by the tissues decreases as the flow increases. The changes in blood oxygen in different areas are contrasted against each other in a process called *blood-oxygen-level dependent* (*BOLD*) contrast imaging. This is a measure of localized brain metabolic activity, which is an indirect way of measuring the electrical activity in specific areas.

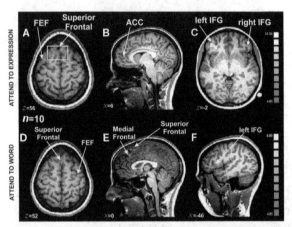

Figure 6.5 Functional Magnetic Resonance Imaging (fMRI) measures changes in blood flow produced by changing metabolic activity. It provides excellent three dimensional geographical isolation of a signal, and good temporal resolution.

its current use for metabolic studies, because fMRI has a much faster time resolution. However, PET can be used with any radioactive tracer; many neurotransmitters and drugs can be made to pinpoint exact locations of neurotransmitter release (with a spatial resolution of millimeters). This is not possible with fMRI.

fMRI measures metabolic hotspots based on measuring changes in the oxygen content of the blood (see Figure 6.5). The microcirculation of blood in the brain is very sensitive to metabolism; an increase in metabolic activity in a region causes vasorelaxation to increase blood flow. However, the increase in blood flow is greater

fMRI combines the millimeter spatial resolution of PET with a relatively rapid temporal resolution (hundreds of milliseconds). One drawback to this method is that changes in blood flow lag behind changes in metabolic activity. This needs to be accounted for in the analysis. Also, the method is limited to blood flow measurements (as opposed to PET's ability to measure neuropharmacological targets).

Diffusion tensor imaging (*DTI*), also called *diffusion tensor tractography*, is an MRI imaging process that detects the movement of water molecules through the axons of the white matter. Myelination makes water stay in the axons rather than diffuse out, which confines random movement of water to up and down the axon. The MRI detects this movement, and computers are used to generate the image. This is used to produce accurate representations of the axonal connections in the brain (see Figure 6.6).

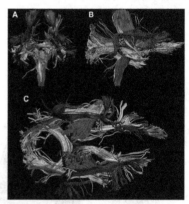

Figure 6.6 Diffusion tensor imaging (DTI) is an MRI imaging process that detects the movement of water molecules through the axons of the white matter. It is used to provide detailed mapping of axonal connections in the brain.

Each of these methods has strengths and weaknesses. The best studies are those that simultaneously record using two or more of these methods and take advantage of the strengths of each.

Three Networks of Cognition
Brain Geography

Each of the three networks discussed here involves interactions between geographically distinct regions of the brain, mainly in the cerebral cortex. Each of the regions is referred to based on where

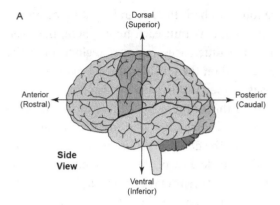

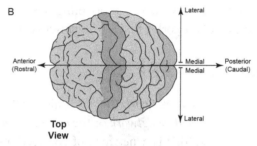

Figure 6.7 A. Two major axes of the brain are front to back (anterior vs. posterior) and top to bottom (dorsal vs. ventral). B. A third axis of the brain is left to right. Because of the bilateral symmetry of the brain, the middle to outside (medial vs. lateral) of each hemisphere are designated.

it lies in the cortex. As discussed in Chapter 4, the cortex is divided into four lobes: frontal, parietal, temporal, and occipital (see Figure 4.12). In addition, the cingulate region is a semicircular structure located inside the lobes of the cortex, closely associated with the limbic system (see Figure 4.11).

In addition to defining these large regions, more specificity is provided by designating three axes of symmetry within the brain (see Figure 6.7). One axis differentiates the front of the brain, which can be called anterior, frontal, or rostral, and the back of the brain, which is called posterior or caudal. This axis is usually designated anterior-posterior. The axis from the top to the bottom of the brain is designated dorsal (or superior, the top) versus ventral (or inferior, the bottom). The third axis is left and right. Typically, similar structures are found in both the left and right hemispheres of the brain. Within each hemisphere, however, there are differences between regions near the center and on the outside. Thus, a medial-lateral axis is defined within each hemisphere.

With this in mind, specific areas in the brain are referred to by their lobe and their position in that lobe. The dorsolateral prefrontal cortex is the upper, outside area of the prefrontal cortex. The ventromedial prefrontal cortex is the lower middle region of the same lobe. While initially confusing, this system is very helpful in orienting oneself to the region of the cortex that is being discussed.

Task-Positive Network

The *task-positive network* (*TPN*) is also called the *central executive network* or the *dorsal attention network*. This is a network of connections between the dorsolateral prefrontal cortex (DLPC) and the posterior parietal cortex (PPC; see Figure 6.8). These regions are active when a person is engaged in an activity that requires focused attention. External information (especially visual) is received. This is processed within working memory, and goal-directed activity is initiated. This is very hard work; it takes effort to activate and sustain this focused attention. Because externally motivated, goal-directed activity can involve all the senses, different cortical regions and networks can become active, depending on the task. However, the core regions of the DLPC and PPC coordinate the cognition.

The prefrontal cortex (PFC) is the most evolutionarily recent area of the brain, being most developed in humans, and the last to be developmentally completed in humans (by around age twenty-six). It is the center of executive functioning, which means that it is the center for foresight, planning, and working memory. This

is higher-order thinking and is required in new situations that haven't been previously practiced.

The DLPC is also the center of cognitive flexibility. *Cognitive flexibility* is holding two different ideas in working memory at the same time and comparing and contrasting them to solving problems. F. Scott Fitzgerald said, "The test of a first-rate intelligence is the ability to hold two opposed ideas in mind at the same time and still retain the ability to function." This decision-making process is a key function of the DLPC, especially in terms of moral and risk-taking behavior.

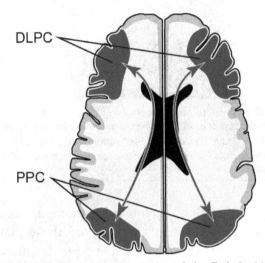

Figure 6.8 The two major nodes of the Task Positive Network (TPN) are the dorsolateral prefrontal cortex (DLPC) and the posterior parietal cortex (PPC).

The PPC receives secondary sensory information from the visual, auditory, and somatosensory cortices. It processes this information to orient a person in space and sends this information to the DLPC. It is very important in attention-requiring activities, as it focuses the DLPC on incoming external and internal stimuli. Together the DLPC and PPC determine a person's physical orientation in the world and decides on actions (i.e., motor neuron output) to perform a task.

The TPN is most actively engaged when a person is totally engrossed in an activity. This is often called being in the "flow state," or being lost in your work. When athletes experience the flow state, they are said to be "in the zone." All attention is focused on incoming stimuli and responding to it. Peripheral, self-referential thoughts are suppressed. Entering and maintaining this focused state can be difficult for some, and it requires mental work to maintain.

Default-Mode Network

When PET became available, many studies were done to determine the parts of the brain utilized by specific tasks. Studies like these helped delineate the cortical regions involved in the TPN. To see which areas were activated during TPN engagement, baseline measurements in a relaxed, unfocused state were first recorded. These were subtracted from the measurements made while performing tasks to identify regions of the cortex that increased in activity during the task.

In the late 1990s, Gordon Shulman did a meta-analysis of nine different previously published PET studies. He noticed that certain areas in the basal state brain *decreased* in activity during TPN activation. That is, certain regions of the brain were more active under rest conditions than they were when actively performing a task. This comparison showed that activating the brain for a specific task not only recruited new parts of the brain from some basal state; it also switched other areas off. This suggested that the brain doesn't just "turn on" during focused activity; it switches from one active mode of thinking to another. This basal activity was called the *default mode*.

The areas of the brain and pathways involved in this relaxed, passive mode of thinking are called the *default-mode network* (*DMN*). The main regions of the brain involved in the DMN are the medial prefrontal cortex (MPC), the posterior cingulate cortex (PCC) and precuneus, and regions of the lateral parietal lobe (LPL; see Figure 6.9).

The dorsal part of the MPC, being part of the PFC, is involved in executive decision making. However, unlike the DLPC of the TPN, the dorsal MPC is involved with self-referential thinking rather than thinking about external stimuli.

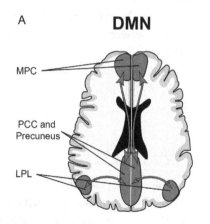
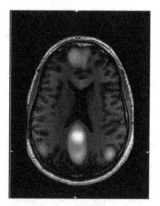

Figure 6.9 A. The three major nodes of the Default Mode Network (DMN) are the medial prefrontal cortex (MPC), the posterior cingulate cortex (PCC), and precuneus and the lateral parietal lobe (LPL). B. fMRI imaging of the active Default Mode Network.

Rather than orienting the person in the physical world, it puts the person into a social context with those around him or her. Future plans are made in this social context.

The dorsal portion of the MPC is active when a person is trying to read the mental state of someone else. This is called *theory of mind*; it is the realization that the other person is distinct from the self, the environment, and other people. Other people are different from a chair, for example, in that they have thoughts like our own. These other people are similar to but separate from the self. (This will have important implications in Chapter 11, when we will be discussing serotonin-like hallucinogens.)

The ventral MPC is important in emotional processing. It forms connections between the senses and the hypothalamus, amygdala, and periaqueductal gray matter. This connects external stimuli and how the stimuli make a person feel (e.g., you see an attractive person, your heart races, your stomach feels fluttery, and your palms sweat). This is important in mood and motivation directed from external cues. This connection between the emotional parts of the brain and the cortex is overactive in depressed people, as will be discussed below.

The PCC and precuneus, along with areas in the LPL, are storage and retrieving areas for self-referential, long-term memories. This includes both spatial memories (putting yourself in a time and place) and autobiographical memories (self-consciousness: "this is who I am"). The spatial memories, in addition to locating where you are now, are part of your cortex's sense of time passing. The DMN does this in coordination with the basal ganglia and cerebellum (timing is crucial to movement). For autobiographical memories, emotional salience is very important to strengthening the connections in this region. Memories that have strong emotions attached to them are stored long term, are easily retrieved, and have a greater impact on personality. The PCC is especially active during mind wandering. It brings up memories of the past and brings them to the attention of the MPC for contextual processing (how does this relate to what has happened before?).

The PCC has connections to the hippocampus that strengthen throughout a typical day. This is how the PCC recalls events of the day, sending these short-term memories to the MPC for conscious awareness. These connections reset to a low level overnight as important (emotionally salient) memories are moved from the hippocampus to the cortex for long-term storage. It is suggested that the PCC may be involved in measuring emotional salience, sending important information to long-term storage in the cortex, and resetting (erasing) the hippocampus during sleep. (This will have important implications in Chapter 10 on cannabis.)

The DMN is crucial to the development of personality. It includes areas of the brain involved in a sense of self (who am I?), a theory of mind (others have a self, too), and orienting the self in social contexts as well as a time and a place. It is active when a person is remembering past events and planning for the future. It is important in social networking; it is the pathway by which people reflect on themselves in their social environment and how to negotiate the best outcomes in their community. It is the introspective part of consciousness.

Salience Network

As its name suggests, the role of the salience network (SN) is to determine what is most important (this was discussed briefly in Chapter 5). It links the DMN and TPN cortical networks to the limbic system emotional network. Its main areas

Imagine that you are riding down the interstate on a long trip, not paying much attention. You don't even notice the landmarks you pass. Ten, twenty minutes go by while you listen to music, think about old relationships, make future plans—anything to take your mind off of the boredom of the road. You look at the mile marker, calculate how much farther you have to go, and estimate how long it will take at your current speed. You hope that there will not be any more road construction like there was one hundred miles back that brought you to a crawl for a half-hour. Default-mode network is your main mode, and ideas are bouncing around your mind like a monkey.

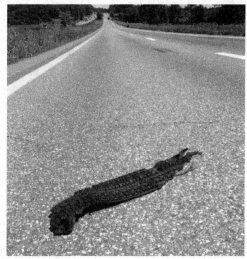

Figure 6.11

Suddenly your awareness is brought to a problem. There is something on the road a short distance ahead, lined up with your left tire. Your SN picks this up, and notes that there is something seriously wrong here. The highway should be clear, and here is something in the way. It quickly switches your thinking over to TPN. TPN tries to identify the object by comparing its size, shape, and color to past experiences (Animal? Garbage? Rock? Sharp? Hard?). Simultaneously, it calculates possible solutions to the problem based on the identity of the object. If it is soft (like a paper bag), hitting it would be safer than swerving. If it is hard or sharp, you will need to swerve around it. As the milliseconds tick off, you decide you won't be able to identify it in time and therefore need to go around it. More decisions. Should you swerve to the right and go around it or left and straddle it? This depends on how high it is and if there is a car in the next lane. Rather than look around, you consult your working memory and recall that there is a car on your right, slightly behind you. You shouldn't swerve in his direction if you don't have to. You decide it is low enough and the safest option is to swerve left and straddle the object. As you fly over it, you notice that it is a torn chunk of a truck tire, and it disappears behind you. All of these calculations and your final correct solution occur in less than one second.

With the problem behind you and the way ahead clear, your SN shifts you back into default mode. You reflect on how quickly all of that happened and marvel at the amazing ability of your mind to analyze a problem and react correctly to it. You think about how it could have gone wrong if it was something big and hard and it blew out your tire. And you plan to write about this experience sometime in the future as a teaching exercise for your students.

are the insular cortex (or insula) and the anterior portion of the cingulate cortex (see Figure 6.10). The *insula* is an area of cortex underneath the parietal cortex in either hemisphere of the brain. It has strong reciprocal connections to the limbic system and to internal and external sensory

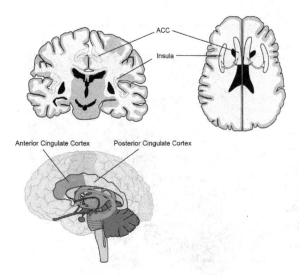

Figure 6.10 The two major nodes of the Salience Network (SN) are the insula and the anterior cingulate cortex (ACC).

organs; it coordinates these inputs to determine a person's emotional state. It is also important for *empathy*, which is changing one's emotional state to match the perception of another person's emotional state.

The other main area in the SN is the *anterior cingulate cortex* (*ACC*). This area is a decision-making area, especially for socially driven interactions. Closely connected to the insula, the ACC checks the emotional state and determines if it is appropriate for what is going on around the person. Based on this error checking, it determines the appropriate network (DMN vs. TPN) to activate.

With this in mind, the SN receives sensory information from both the external world and the internal environment. If external cues are out of the norm (e.g., your car has drifted across the dividing line), the SN brings this to conscious awareness (i.e., the SN activates the TPN). If the external cues align with what's expected, the SN allows consciousness to relax in default mode (DMN). This is error detection; if things are out of balance, it activates the network needed to react to the event.

The reaction can be based on an emotional need (e.g., hunger, emotional distress, or cravings) or external stimuli. In this capacity, the SN acts as a central hub between the sensory awareness of the world and internal states and the two main cognitive networks, the TPN and DMN. It controls the balance between these two networks.

Integration

In a neurotypical individual, the DMN and TPN networks are seamlessly integrated (see Box 6.1 and Figure 6.12). The brain unconsciously switches between them as needed based on external and internal cues received. There is an "anti-correlation" between the DMN and TPN pathways, that is, between externally focused and unfocused states. As focused attention is needed, the TPN is activated and the DMN become quieter; introspection is repressed, and because the DMN is important for sensing the passage of time, a person loses himself in a task and time seems to pass quickly. As a person becomes more introspective, the TPN grows quieter and DMN is active. When a person is bored (with no task

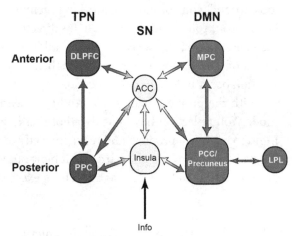

Figure 6.12 Normal connectivity shows a balance within and between networks, with the Salience Network (SN) controlling the flow of information between networks.

to perform), the person is continually in default mode; time seems to pass very slowly because one is more aware of its passing. When self-referential thinking intrudes on a task, maintaining focus becomes difficult. Internal sensing (e.g., nausea, the need to urinate/defecate, pain, or fatigue) activates DMN, making it hard to focus on a task. Emotionally stressful situations (e.g., anxiety) increase activity in the DMN, also making it difficult to focus. Brain development, especially in the critical years between ten and thirteen years of age, is associated with the development of greater connectivity within the DMN and TPN and greater separation between them.

However, these two pathways are not mutually exclusive. Many tasks, especially creative tasks, switch rapidly back and forth between the two states or activate both at the same time. Indeed, creativity is thought to involve accessing the DMN while simultaneously performing a task with TPN. The strengths and skills of each network can be recruited.

Cognitive Disorders

The understanding of different modes of thinking may help explain many of the symptoms seen in cognitive disorders and the underlying alteration in information processing. It also helps explain altered modes of consciousness produced by drugs, especially hallucinogens. The important changes in cognitive disorders tend to be connectivity problems within a network and between networks. When this breaks down, cognition suffers.

The descriptions below are not meant to be comprehensive explanations of the disorders discussed. These are brief outlines of current research into three cognitive disorders to provide a context for how cognition works and what

happens when the functional connectivity of the systems is not neurotypical. Also, within each of these conditions there is much variation; the descriptions may not apply to everyone who has been diagnosed with the disorder.

Depression

Depression is a common, debilitating disorder that affects approximately 6.7% of the U.S. population. Depression is characterized by excessive rumination on negative thoughts, impaired ability to direct attention outward, and hypersensitivity to negative thought initiation. People with depression are unable to move away from negative thoughts and feelings and reorient toward positive activities, such as goal-directed task completion. The result is obsession with negative, self-referential thoughts, and an inability to function normally.

fMRI studies suggest that a central problem in depression may be a deficiency in the ACC's ability to switch away from DMN and into TPN (see Figure 6.13). The MPC is connected

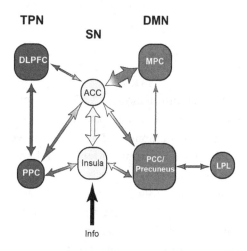

Figure 6.13 In depression, there is a stronger connection between the ACC and the MPC, directing excessive cognitive processing towards self-rumination. There is also a weakened connection within the DMN.

through the ACC to the limbic system, especially the amygdala. In depression, the connection between the MPC and limbic system (between thought and emotion) predominates cognition and is difficult to break. Normally, the SN turns down the DMN as it activates the TPN, and the TPN exerts "top-down" control over the limbic system, squelching emotions in favor of completing a task. In other words, a non-depressed person may decide, "I'll think about that later. Right now I need to get work done." A depressed person with diminished ACC function has difficulty making this switch, remains stuck in negative, self-involved thought patterns, and is unable to function normally.

In addition, a decreased linkage between the anterior part of the DMN (MPC) and the posterior parts (PCC and precuneus) has been seen in depressed people. This suggests that the negative thought patterns are unrealistic, in that they are not tied to the parts of the brain that establish self-identity. This is a dissociation, of sorts, between a previously established sense of self and emotionally driven, overly negative rumination on the self.

Autism

Autism spectrum disorder (ASD) is a developmental disorder characterized by deficiencies in social development and interaction, verbal and nonverbal communication, and behavior. ASD symptoms can vary from mild to severe. Individuals with ASD vary in the severity of the expression in each of these three areas, but all exhibit some deficiency in each.

Many recent studies have been conducted to determine changes in the functional connectivity within and between the three major cognitive networks, often with conflicting results. This may

be due to developmental differences between subjects or between methodologies to measure connectivity. However, comprehensive studies of all three cognitive networks have determined some commonalities in ASD.

The most consistent result of these studies is the discovery of reduced functional connectivity between the frontal and posterior areas of the DMN (see Figure 6.14). This connection between the MPC and the PCC/precuneus is important in the theory of mind processing (I am someone, and so are you). The loss of connectivity in the DMN may underlie the difficulties in social interactions.

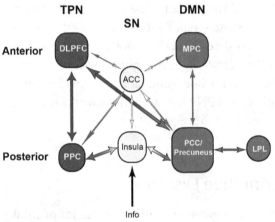

Figure 6.14 ASD seems to arise from several problems in cognition. There is underconnectivity between the anterior and posterior nodes of the DMN and between the insula and the ACC of the SN. There is also commonly overconnectivity between the PCC of the DMN and the DLPC of the TPN, which should segregate during development.

Another important finding is under-connectivity within the SN, which correlates directly with impairments in social communication. Recall that the insula is responsible for determining a person's emotional state and for empathizing with others' emotional states. The ACC performs error detection on this input, that is, determines whether these emotional states are correct. This lack of functional connectivity between these two regions of the SN results in difficulties in social connection between one's own emotional state and that of others. This is commonly expressed by an autistic person's inability to understand the emotional states of others.

Another consequence of this decreased connectivity between the insula and ACC is an impaired hub function. The SN normally switches between TPN and DMN based on emotional and external cues. The lack of this hub function makes transitions between focused attention and relaxed states difficult.

In addition, persons with ASD have overconnectivity between their PCC (part of the DMN) and their DLPC (part of the TPN), especially on the right side of the brain. This cross-connectivity inhibits the anti-correlation between the DMN and TPN in neurotypical individuals. As a result, the normal shutting off of the DMN during focused task activity is weakened, and the person has difficulty focusing on a task. This is a reduction in the typical segregation between networks that is vital to cognition.

Thus, ASD is characterized by network-specific connectivity problems—overconnectivity between some regions (between PCC and DLPC) and under-connectivity between others (within the insula and ACC in the SN). These connectivity issues produce the social, communicative, and behavioral problems seen in ASD.

Attention Deficient Hyperactivity Disorder

Attention deficient hyperactivity disorder (ADHD) is a developmental disorder of cognitive processing. People with this problem have difficulty maintaining focused attention on a task, tend to be overactive, and have difficulty controlling their behavior. The developmental nature of this disorder is seen in the fact that this type of behavior is normal for small children (about five to six years old) but typically declines in children with age. People with ADHD have difficulty focusing and controlling their behavior into adulthood. In general, the normal developmental strengthening within the three cognitive networks and segregation between them does not occur to the same extent in ADHD.

People with ADHD have attention lapses and the intrusion of self-referential thinking during task performance, which makes staying focused difficult. This suggests that there is a problem in the SN's allocation of attentional resources, and this is what is seen in ADHD (see Figure 6.15). In normally developing children, the functional connectivity between the ACC of the SN and the PCC of the DMN declines with age; this relates to the developmental segregation between these two networks. In people with ADHD, this connection

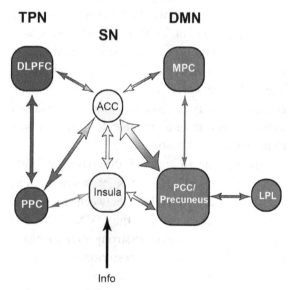

Figure 6.15 In ADHD, the functional connectivity between the ACC of the SN and the PCC of the DMN, which should normally decline with age, remains strong. In addition there is an abnormally weak connection between insula of the SN and PPC of TPN. Finally, there is a lack of strengthening between the anterior and posterior nodes of the DMN.

Table 6.1

TPN	DLPC	Executive Control (Tasks) Foresight & Planning (Tasks) Cognitive Flexibility	Focused Attention on Task Flow State
	PPC	Orientation in space Learned Movements	
DMN	MPC	Executive Control (Self) Foresight & Planning (Tasks)	Mind wandering Self-referential thoughts (Introspection) Development of Personality Social Awareness
	Precuneus, PCC & LPC	Theory of Mind Emotional Processing Self-referential long-term memories Emotional Salience	
SN	Insula	Coordinate emotions Empathy	Central Hub Directs awareness to either TPN or DMN
	ACC	Emotional Error Checking Decision making	

stays abnormally strong. In addition, there is an abnormally weak connection between insula of the SN and PPC of TPN. This results in a lack of anti-correlation between the TPN and DMN, which is seen in typically developing children. These changes correlate to behavioral problems and the inability to maintain focused attention, as the SN is unable to adequately shift attention to the necessary network.

Another developmental difference in children with ADHD is a lack of strengthening of functional connections between the MPC and the posterior parts of the DMN (PCC and precuneus). Thus, there are stronger connections between the SN and the posterior positions of the DMN, but weaker connections between this and the executive control areas of the DMN. The tighter the connections within the DMN are, the more mature the resource allocation system is and the higher the IQ.

Overall, people with ADHD lack the common developmentally acquired segregation between cognitive networks and strengthening within them. Connection between the ACC and the posterior portion of the DMN fail to weaken with age, while the connections between the insula and the TPN fail to strengthen. Also, the inter-network connections between the anterior and posterior parts of the DMN fail to strengthen. This developmental delay makes focused task activities very difficult for people with ADHD.

Summary

Cognition involves rapid integration of many different factors. Sensory information enters into consciousness from internal sources (physical and emotional sensing) and external sources (visual, auditory, somatosensory, etc.). This is put into the context of who the person is in time (the "now" coordinated with past experiences and future plans) and space. Decisions on actions are made based on error detection between current conditions and expectations. This exquisitely tuned processing is performed by the separation of tasks into distinct anatomical regions of the brain connected by networks of axons. The TPN, whose central regions are the DLPC and the PPC, is active during externally focused task performance. The DMN, located in the MPC, PCC, precuneus, and LPL, coordinates the rest state of consciousness. It synthesizes the sense of self from past experiences, future plans, and social contexts. It also controls the sense of time passing. Located both physically and functionally between these two networks is the SN. It is composed of the insula and ACC. Its function is to detect internal and external sensory information, decide if this is normal or not, and direct attention toward the TPN or the DMN, depending on which is most important at the time. Developmental maturation involves strengthening connections within each of these networks and segregation between them. When these networks are not properly strengthened, segregated, and integrated, cognitive dysfunction such as depression, ASD, and ADHD may develop.

Further Reading

Brain imaging: Bonifacio, G., and G. Zamboni. "Brain Imaging in Dementia." *Postgraduate Medical Journal* 92 (2016): 333–40.

Buckner, R. L., F. M. Krienen, and B. T. T. Yeo. "Opportunities and Limitations of Intrinsic Functional Connectivity MRI." *Nature Neuroscience* 16 (2013): 832–7.

Dennis, E. L., and P. M. Thompson. "Functional Brain Connectivity Using fMRI in Aging and Alzheimer's Disease." *Neuropsychology Review* 24 (2014): 49–62.

Brain networks: Bressler, S. L., and V. Menon. "Large-Scale Brain Networks in Cognition: Emerging Methods and Principles." *Trends in Cognitive Sciences* 14 (2010): 277–90.

Default-mode network: Raichle, M. E. "The Brain's Default Mode Network." *Annual Review of Neuroscience* 38 (2015): 433–47.

Shulman, G. L., J. A. Fiez, M. Corbetta, R. L. Buckner, F. M. Miezen, M. E. Raichle, and S. E. Peterseb. "Common Blood Flow Changes across Visual Tasks: Decreases in Cerebral Cortex." *Journal of Cognitive Neuroscience* 9 (1997): 648–63.

Salience network: Uddin, Lucina Q. "Salience Processing and Insular Cortical Function and Dysfunction." *Nature Reviews Neuroscience* 16 (2015): 55–61.

DMN and depression: Marchetti, I., E. H. W. Koster, E. J. Sonuga-Barke, and R. De Raedt. "The Default Mode Network and Recurrent Depression: A Neurobiological Model of Cognitive Risk Factors." *Neuropsychology Reviews* 22 (2012): 229–51.

ASD: Abbott, A. E., A. Nair, C. L. Keown, M. Datko, A. Jahedi, I. Fishman, and R. A. Müller. "Patterns of Atypical Functional Connectivity and Behavioral Links in Autism Differ Between Default, Salience, and Executive Networks." *Cerebral Cortex* 26 (2015): 4034–45.

ADHD: Choi, J., B. Jeong, S. W. Lee, and H. J. Gol. "Aberrant Development of Functional Connectivity among Resting State-Related Functional Networks in Medication-Naive ADHD Children." *PLOS One* 8 (2013): 1–12.

Test Your Understanding
Multiple-Choice

1. This method of measuring activity in the brain produces the fastest three-dimensional recordings:
   a. EEG
   b. MEG
   c. PET
   d. fMRI
2. The distinction between the top of your brain and the bottom is
   a. anterior-posterior
   b. dorsal-ventral
   c. medial-lateral
   d. rostral-caudal
3. The cingulate cortex is functionally divided into two parts. The ACC is part of the _____ and the PCC is part of the _____.
   a. DMN, TPN
   b. TPN, DMN
   c. SN, TPN
   d. SN, DMN
4. The most anterior portion of the DMN is the
   a. MPC
   b. DLPC
   c. LPL
   d. PPC
5. The TPN is composed of the
   a. DLPC and the PCC
   b. MPC and the LPL
   c. DLPC and the PPC
   d. MPC and the PCC
6. This part of the SN determines your emotional state and is important for empathy:
   a. insula
   b. ACC
   c. PCC
   d. LPL

7. This part of the DMN is important for the sense of self that organizes your personality:
   a. MPC
   b. PPC
   c. precuneus
   d. PCC
8. One functional change in depression is
   a. overconnectivity between the PCC and DLPC
   b. a hyperactive limbic to MPC connection
   c. a weakened connection between the ACC and MPC
   d. all of the above

Essay Questions

1. What are the strengths and weakness of EEG as a means of measuring brain activity?
2. What is the role of the salience network (SN)?
3. When a person is very focused on a task, we often say they are in a flow state, or in the zone. Explain this in terms of the task-positive network (TPN) and the default-mode network (DMN) and the anti-correlation between the two. How does TPN lead one to lose sense of self and time?
4. What would happen if a person lost the connection between the anterior and posterior regions of the DMN?
5. What is the developmental problem that occurs in ADHD in terms of the three cognitive networks? What symptoms does this produce?

Credits

- Fig. 6.0: Copyright © 2014 by Andreashorn / Wikimedia Commons, (CC BY-SA 4.0) at https://commons.wikimedia.org/wiki/File:Default_Mode_Network_Connectivity.png.
- Fig. 6.2a: Antoine Lutz / Copyright in the Public Domain.
- Fig. 6.2b: Copyright © 2012 by Otoomuch / Wikimedia Commons, (CC BY-SA 3.0) at https://commons.wikimedia.org/wiki/File:EEG_Closing_eyes.png.
- Fig. 6.3: National Institutes of Health / Copyright in the Public Domain.
- Fig. 6.4a: Kieran Maher / Copyright in the Public Domain.
- Fig. 6.4b: National Institutes of Health / Copyright in the Public Domain.
- Fig. 6.5: Copyright © 2010 by Shima Ovaysikia, Khalid A. Tahir, Jason L. Chan, and Joseph F. X. DeSouza, (CC BY 2.5) at https://commons.wikimedia.org/wiki/File:FMRI_BOLD_activation_in_an_emotional_Stroop_task.jpg.
- Fig. 6.6: Copyright © 2015 by Roine, et al., (CC BY-SA 4.0) at https://commons.wikimedia.org/wiki/File:Tractography_from_the_diffusion_weighted_data.jpg.
- Fig. 6.9b: John Graner / Copyright in the Public Domain.

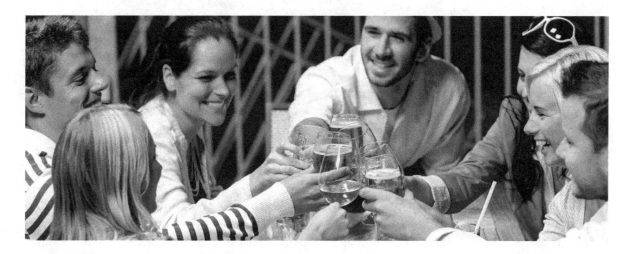

Chapter 7: Alcohol

Introduction

Alcohol is a drug that had been consumed recreationally by animals long before humans evolved. Many species of birds and mammals today, including most primates, are known to eat rotten fruit specifically for the alcohol it contains and become inebriated. It is probably safe to say that humans have consumed alcohol as long as we have existed. Alcohol is the second most widely used drug today, behind caffeine. It is also considered the most destructive drug worldwide because of its wide availability and potential for chronic abuse.

What we call "alcohol" is more specifically called *ethanol* or *ethyl alcohol*. Many other forms of alcohol exist that vary in their structure from ethyl alcohol, some of which we encounter regularly in the home (see Figure 7.1). Methyl or wood alcohol is often used as a solvent for degreasing. This is sometimes drunk, usually by mistake, and is very toxic. It causes blindness, coma, and even death. Methanol is often added to ethanol to make

the ethanol undrinkable and allow for its commercial sale, for example, at the hardware store.

Figure 7.1 Any organic chemical with a hydroxyl group (-OH) is categorized as an alcohol. Examples are methyl alcohol (wood alcohol), ethyl alcohol, and isopropyl alcohol (rubbing alcohol).

Isopropanol (rubbing alcohol) is also in common household use. This is an effective disinfectant often used to clean a wound or the skin before a hypodermic injection. Isopropanol is also highly toxic and not for internal use.

Ethyl alcohol is most commonly produced by the anaerobic fermentation of sugars by bacteria or yeast. Any sugars will do; wheat, barley, corn, grape juice, apple cider, sugar cane, and many other sources of sugar are used to produce it. The concentration that can be achieved by bacteria or yeast is limited to approximately 15 to 20%; at this point the alcohol becomes toxic to the organism and fermentation stops. To get a higher concentration of ethanol, it is separated from water by the process of distillation. Distillation can achieve

95% ethanol, and further purification is possible only through more complicated chemical techniques.

Alcoholic beverages can be found in a number of forms related to taste preferences among the consumers (see Figure 7.2). Beer is made by fermenting malted barley (barley that has been allowed to germinate) and is flavored by using different types and treatments of the barley and by adding the flowers of the hop plant. Light beers are approximately 3% alcohol, and stronger beers can reach 10% or greater. Wine is made by fermenting different varieties of grapes (e.g., merlot, cabernet, or pinot grapes) with various strains of yeast and is typically between 10% and 16% alcohol.

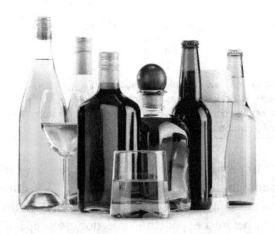

Figure 7.2 Alcohol can be purchased in a number of different forms. Among these is wine, cordials or liqueurs, distilled spirits (whiskeys, rum, etc.), and beers.

Stronger drinks are made with distilled alcohol. Cordials and liqueurs are strong, sweet drinks that are made by adding fruit, nuts, and/or spices to distilled alcohol. The alcohol concentration is designed into the making of the drink and is typically from 15 to 50%. Spirits, or hard liquor, are similar to liqueurs, except no sugar is added. Flavors are added to the distillate and

it is diluted to the proper alcohol concentration (usually 40% or 46%); it may then be aged in barrels to enhance flavors. Whiskey, gin, tequila, rum, and vodka, among others, are made this way and are distinguished by their fermentation source and flavorings added after distillation. The concentration of alcohol in spirits is usually designated by the term *proof*, which is twice the alcohol concentration (thus, 40% alcohol is 80 proof). This is a designation that originated with British sailors, who would test their daily rum allotment by soaking gunpowder in it. If the gunpowder could still be lit, this was 100 proof—that is, it was not watered down.

Pharmacokinetics

Alcohol is almost always taken orally. This is for cultural reasons and because drinks are designed to taste good as well as be a delivery method for the drug. However, alcohol can also be volatilized and inhaled or absorbed through mucous membranes.

When taken orally, it is absorbed mainly in the small intestine, with about 10% being absorbed in stomach. The time to the peak concentration in the blood, as well as the peak itself, is variable depending on the amount of food present in the stomach. When taken on an empty stomach, alcohol will peak in the blood in approximately thirty minutes. However, if alcohol is taken on a full stomach, it will peak much more slowly (in as much as ninety minutes) as the contents of the stomach are mixed and slowly released into the small intestine. This has consequences for the peak concentration of alcohol as well. Alcohol is metabolized by the enzyme alcohol dehydrogenase (ADH; see Figure 7.3), which is present in the lining of the stomach. When the alcohol stays longer in the stomach, the ADH metabolizes more of it before it can be absorbed in the small intestine. This represents the first level of first-pass metabolism of alcohol, and it decreases the amount that reaches the blood.

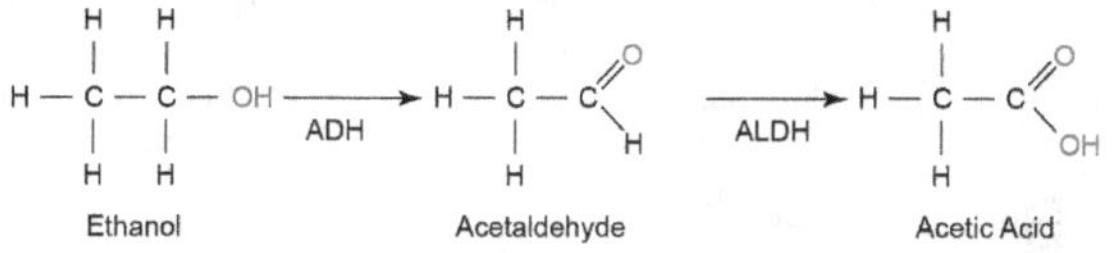

Figure 7.3 Ethanol is first oxidized to acetaldehyde by alcohol dehydrogenase (ADH). This toxic metabolite is then oxidized to the harmless compound acetic acid by the enzyme aldehyde dehydrogenase (ALDH). Acetic acid is then further metabolized for energy or synthesized into fat and stored.

Alcohol is widely distributed throughout the body. Its structure is somewhat polar, and it preferentially partitions into aqueous compartments. However, it is a small molecule and can slip through phospholipid barriers, including the blood-brain barrier.

Ethyl alcohol is metabolized into acetaldehyde by ADH, and acetaldehyde is further metabolized into acetic acid by aldehyde dehydrogenase (ALDH; see Figure 7.3). Acetic acid is a common metabolite in cells and is easily used for energy production or to synthesize fats for storage. The first metabolite, acetaldehyde, on the other hand, produces inflammation and is very toxic to cells. Its production may lead to some of the negative effects of a hangover (see below). The drug disulfiram is sometimes used as aversion therapy in the treatment of alcoholics. It blocks ALDH, causing a buildup of acetaldehyde, and makes the user very uncomfortable. Asian flush syndrome is a condition related to the metabolism of alcohol. A large percentage of Asians (up to 80% of some populations) have a variant of the ADH enzyme that is much more efficient at producing acetaldehyde, which produces a flushing of the skin due to inflammation. This is exacerbated

in some individuals who also have a variant of the ALDH enzyme that is less efficient, allowing acetaldehyde to build up even further.

Most of the alcohol consumed is metabolized (95%), both in the liver (80%) and the stomach (15%). However, a significant amount is eliminated by the kidneys and exhaled from the lungs (the exhaled alcohol is the basis for breathalyzer testing). The metabolism of alcohol is rare among drugs in that it follows zero-order kinetics (see Figure 1.12B), meaning that it is removed from the blood at a constant rate. This is because a large amount of alcohol is consumed compared to other drugs for a similar effect (e.g., two drinks has 20 grams of alcohol, which is equivalent to 2 milligrams of diazepam). At this concentration, the enzyme ADH is saturated, metabolizing the alcohol as fast as it is able. This results in a constant rate of metabolism until most of the alcohol is removed. This rate is approximately one drink per hour (12 ounces of 5% beer, 6 ounces of wine, or 1.5 ounces of spirits).

Blood alcohol content (BAC) is the commonly used measure of alcohol in the body. The BAC produced by an amount of ingested alcohol can be estimated using sex and body weight as an approximate guide (see Figure 7.4), although it varies based on a number of factors. The speed of drinking can affect BAC. Drinking at a slow rate allows metabolism to catch up to consumption. Having one drink per hour should result in a constant BAC over time. Stomach contents can affect BAC because they affect absorption rate and metabolism, as described above. A person's size also affects BAC; a larger person has a greater volume in which to dilute the alcohol (see Figure 7.5A), lowering the BAC for the same amount of alcohol. This is called the *volume of distribution* of the drug. Another factor in volume of distribution is the percent body fat. Alcohol preferentially partitions into aqueous compartments,

⭐ **Approximate Blood Alcohol Percentage In One Hour For A Woman**

Source: National Highway Traffic Safety Administration

Approximate Blood Alcohol Percentage In One Hour For A Woman

Drinks	Body Weight in Pounds								Influenced
	100	120	140	160	180	200	220	240	
1	.05	.04	.03	.03	.03	.02	.02	.02	Possibly
2	.09	.08	.07	.06	.05	.05	.04	.04	
3	.14	.11	.11	.09	.08	.07	.06	.06	Impaired
4	.18	.15	.13	.11	.10	.09	.08	.08	
5	.23	.19	.16	.14	.13	.11	.10	.09	Legally Intoxicated
6	.27	.23	.19	.17	.15	.14	.12	.11	
7	.32	.27	.23	.20	.18	.16	.14	.13	
8	.36	.30	.26	.23	.20	.18	.17	.15	
9	.41	.34	.29	.26	.23	.20	.19	.17	
10	.45	.38	.32	.28	.25	.23	.21	.19	

⭐ **Approximate Blood Alcohol Percentage In One Hour For A Man**

Source: National Highway Traffic Safety Administration

Approximate Blood Alcohol Percentage In One Hour For A Man

Drinks	Body Weight in Pounds								Influenced
	100	120	140	160	180	200	220	240	
1	.04	.03	.03	.02	.02	.02	.02	.02	Possibly
2	.08	.06	.05	.05	.04	.04	.03	.03	
3	.11	.09	.08	.07	.06	.06	.05	.05	Impaired
4	.15	.12	.11	.09	.08	.08	.07	.06	
5	.19	.16	.13	.12	.11	.09	.09	.08	Legally Intoxicated
6	.23	.19	.16	.14	.13	.11	.10	.09	
7	.26	.22	.19	.16	.15	.13	.12	.11	
8	.30	.25	.21	.19	.17	.15	.14	.13	
9	.34	.28	.24	.21	.19	.17	.15	.14	
10	.38	.31	.27	.23	.21	.19	.17	.16	

Subtract .015 for each hour after drinking.

One drink is based on 1.5 oz. of 80 proof liquor (40%), 12 oz. beer (4.5%), or 5 oz. wine (12%).

Note: The figures are averages and may vary based on the amount of food in your stomach.

Figure 7.4 Blood alcohol concentration can be approximately predicted based on sex and the amount imbibed.

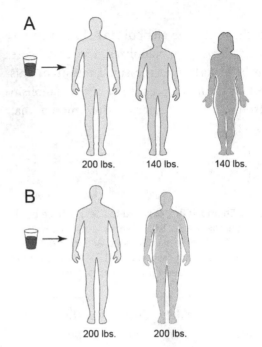

Figure 7.5 A. The volume of distribution of alcohol varies with size as well as sex of the person. (Darker brown represents a higher BAC. Yellow represents fat.) B. The volume of distribution of alcohol varies with the percent of body fat of the person.

so a person with a higher body fat percentage will have a smaller volume of distribution than a person with a lower body fat percentage for the same body mass (see Figure 7.5B), raising the BAC. Carbonation in a drink increases its rate of absorption and increases BAC. This is why people often say champagne goes straight to their heads. And previous exposure can affect BAC. A person who is a frequent consumer of alcohol will have a higher level of ADH than an infrequent user would. This causes more rapid metabolism and a lower BAC for the same amount consumed (more on this in the section on tolerance below).

Another major factor in BAC is sex. Women will normally have a higher BAC than men for the same amount consumed (see Figure 7.4), for several reasons. First, women tend to be smaller in size, which decreases their volume of distribution.

They also have a higher body fat percent, which also decreases volume of distribution (see Figure 7.5A). Women have less ADH in their stomach; this decreases first-pass metabolism and increases absorption. Finally, birth control medication increases the rate of absorption of alcohol, increasing the peak BAC.

Mechanism of Action

Alcohol has two distinct mechanisms of action, depending on the dose. At lower doses, alcohol blocks glutamate receptors, decreases glutamate release, and stimulates GABA receptors (see Figure 7.6). This makes the brain less sensitive to endogenously released glutamate and more sensitive to endogenously released GABA. Glutamate

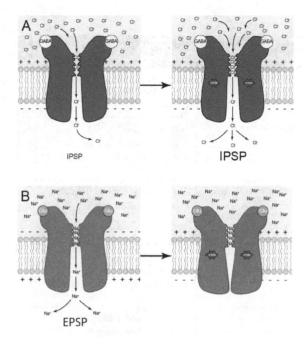

Figure 7.6 A. Alcohol increases the amount of chloride (Cl⁻) entering a cell due to GABA stimulation. B. Alcohol decreases the amount of sodium (Na⁺) entering a cell due to glutamate stimulation.

is an excitatory neurotransmitter, and GABA is an inhibitory neurotransmitter, so the effect of low-dose alcohol on these receptors decreases excitability in the brain. These receptors are important all over the brain, but are especially important in the hippocampus (memory), amygdala (emotion), prefrontal cortex (executive function), and cerebellum (balance and motion). The long-term effect of chronic alcohol abuse is an upregulation of glutamate receptors and a downregulation of GABA receptors. This has serious consequences in withdrawal (see below).

An indirect consequence of these effects on glutamate and GABA receptors is to modulate other neurotransmitters, especially endorphins. Alcohol increases the release of endorphins, which indirectly causes the release of dopamine in the limbic system (see Chapter 8). This stimulates the pleasure center: the nucleus accumbens, dorsal striatum, amygdala, hippocampus, and prefrontal cortex. This why alcohol produces a pleasant, slightly euphoric, relaxing sense of well-being and also why it can be addictive.

The second mechanism of action of alcohol is nonspecific and occurs at high doses. Alcohol, being somewhat nonpolar, dissolves in the plasma membranes of neurons at high concentrations. This disrupts the interactions between the phospholipids, making the membrane more fluid (see Figure 7.7). The function of all membrane proteins will be affected by this, including the receptors and ion channels involved in information processing. The result is a generalized shutdown of neurons and therefore brain function. This is similar to the effect of general anesthetics, such as ether or nitrous oxide.

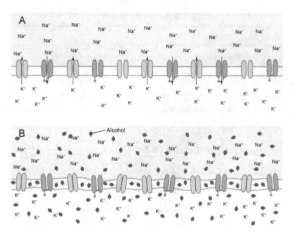

Figure 7.7 A. Normal function of ion channels in the absence of alcohol. B. The function of ion channels is disrupted by the solvent effects of high dose alcohol in the membrane, which makes the membrane more fluid.

Psychological and Physiological Effects
Psychological Effects

Alcohol is classified as a sedative-hypnotic; it decreases anxiety and induces sleep. Effects are dose-dependent, increasing in magnitude as BAC

Progressive Effects of Alcohol

Blood Alcohol Concentration	Changes in Feelings and Personality	Brain Regions Affected	Impaired Activities (continuum)
0.01 -0.05	Relaxation Sense of well being Loss of inhibition	Cerebral cortex	Alertness Judgment Coordination
0.06-0.10	Pleasure Numbing of feelings Nausea, Sleepiness Emotional arousal	Cerebral cortex + forebrain	(especially fine motor skills) Visual tracking Reasoning and depth perception
0.11 -0.20	Mood swings Anger Sadness Mania	Cerebral cortex + forebrain + cerebellum	Inappropriate social behavior (e.g., obnoxiousness)
0.21 -0.30	Aggression Reduced sensations Depression Stupor	Cerebral cortex + forebrain + cerebellum + brain stem	Slurred speech Lack of balance Loss of temperature regulation
0.31-0.40	Unconsciousness Death possible Coma	Entire brain	Loss of bladder control Difficulty breathing
0.41 and greater	Death		Slowed heart rate

Source: Advisory committee and NIAAA scientists.

Figure 7.8 The effects of alcohol are dose-dependent. Low doses are mild and pleasant while high doses lead to vomiting, stupor, and death.

increases (see Figure 7.8). Low doses produce relaxation and a positive mood. At medium doses, muscle control, inhibitions, and reaction times are affected. At high doses, alcohol induces sleep, vomiting, and stupor, and can even cause death.

At low doses, the indirect effect of alcohol on endorphins activates the limbic system, producing a mild euphoria. It also inhibits the prefrontal cortex, decreasing anxiety and reducing inhibitions. The prefrontal cortex normally keeps the emotional part of the brain (the limbic system) in check. As the cortex releases control, the person feels more relaxed and is more likely to act on feelings. This decrease in inhibitions produces greater risk taking and impulsive behavior. In a social setting, the relaxation of inhibitions may make a person more excited, despite the direct inhibitory effect of the drug, and more personable and talkative. On the other hand, it may make the person more aggressive or depressed, depending on the setting and person's natural inclinations.

Another dose-dependent effect of alcohol is the inhibition of the release of antidiuretic hormone from the posterior pituitary. This will be discussed below in the section on peripheral effects.

At higher doses the inhibitory effects increase, and the person becomes less aware of his or her surroundings. Coordination decreases (partially due to effects on the cerebellum), as does reaction time. This makes driving particularly dangerous. The perceived speed of an automobile is underestimated, further decreasing driving competence. The decrease in situational awareness also makes violent, aggressive activity more likely. Half of all convicted violent offenders in federal prison were intoxicated when they committed their offense or had a history of alcohol abuse (http://www.centeronaddiction.org/addiction-research/reports/behind-bars-ii-substance-abuse-and-america%E2%80%99s-prison-population).

At very high doses, the nonspecific effects of the drug cause a general shutdown of brain activity. Memories are no longer saved, and the user experiences "blackouts," or loss of memory while drunk. Coordination is entirely lost, resulting in stumbling, slurring of words, and generally incoherent behavior. This progresses with dose to the point of unconsciousness (stupor), inducing vomiting as well (via the area postrema in the medulla). Respiration is depressed and may cease at high enough concentrations. The combination of vomiting (followed by aspiration of the vomit) and respiratory depression can cause death during extreme alcohol toxicity.

Peripheral Effects

Many studies have shown that moderate daily intake of alcohol has a positive effect on cardiovascular health. One to three drinks per day can decrease the risk of heart attack or stroke from 40 to 60% (see Figure 7.9A). This is probably because of its effects on lipoproteins in the blood. Moderate doses of alcohol increase high-density lipoproteins (HDL, good cholesterol) and decrease low-density lipoproteins (LDL, bad cholesterol). This is good for cardiovascular health because it decreases the likelihood that plaque will form inside arteries (see Figure 7.9B). Plaque narrows arteries and restricts blood flow to the affected tissues; this increases the possibility of a total blockage (thrombosis). Also, vasodilation caused by alcohol increases CNS blood flow, which can decrease dementia in the elderly.

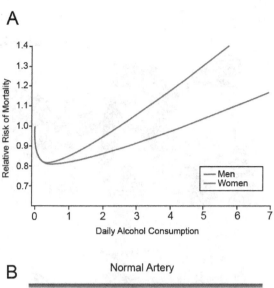

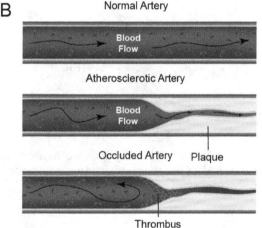

Figure 7.9 A. Moderate consumption of alcohol (1-3 drinks per day) provides protection for adverse cardiovascular events. Higher doses reverse this trend. B. High concentrations of LDL in the blood lead to the formation of plaques, which occlude arteries, restricting blood flow. Plaques also increase the likelihood of thrombosis, or total blockage of the artery.

However, with heavy use, the good effects diminish and are replaced by cardiovascular failure, liver damage, and increased cancer of the mouth, esophagus, stomach, and liver.

Another peripheral effect, which is initiated centrally, is dehydration caused by diuresis in the kidneys. This is caused by the inhibition of the release of antidiuretic hormone from the

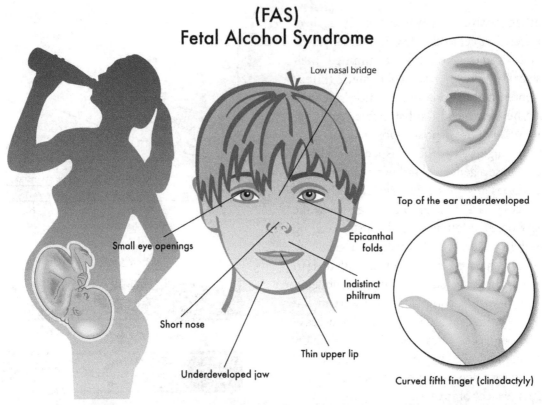

(FAS)
Fetal Alcohol Syndrome

Low nasal bridge

Top of the ear underdeveloped

Small eye openings

Epicanthal folds

Indistinct philtrum

Short nose

Thin upper lip

Underdeveloped jaw

Curved fifth finger (clinodactyly)

Figure 7.10 The most obvious symptoms of a child or adult with FAS are facial deformities: short nose, flat philtrum, thin upper lip, folds of skin above eyes, and underdeveloped jaw, and small eye openings.

posterior pituitary. Caffeine, another diuretic that is often taken along with alcohol, magnifies this effect. Dehydration produces some of the symptoms referred to as a "hangover," discussed below. In addition, diuresis causes a rapid loss of water-soluble vitamins (e.g., C and B1); this can be exacerbated in chronic alcoholics and causes metabolic deficiencies.

Teratogenic Effects

Alcohol produces birth defects when taken at high doses during pregnancy. The most extreme form of this is called fetal alcohol syndrome (FAS), which is seen in 30 to 50% of births to alcoholic mothers. The risk of having a child with FAS is higher in women who drink early in pregnancy, who drink larger amounts more often, and who have other compounding factors such as poor nutrition, cigarette smoking, or a lack of prenatal care.

The most obvious symptoms of a child or adult with FAS are facial deformities (see Figure 7.10): short nose, flat philtrum and thin upper lip, folds of skin above the eyes, an underdeveloped jaw, and small eye openings. Common CNS problems are more disturbing. Children with FAS have developmental delays, are at risk of attention deficit hyperactivity disorder (ADHD), and have attachment issues. Adults tend to not make the connection between their actions and future events, which suggests underdevelopment of the prefrontal cortex. They tend to lack social skills, abuse drugs and alcohol, and have difficulty maintaining employment. These traits, combined with antisocial behavior that is common in FAS adults, make them likely to end up in the criminal justice system.

Other milder forms of this syndrome include partial fetal alcohol syndrome (pFAS) and alcohol-related neurodevelopmental disorder (ARND). These are less severe forms of the syndrome but are more common.

Tolerance and Dependence
Types of Tolerance

Tolerance occurs when the body responds to a substance to minimize its effects. When a person becomes tolerant to alcohol, its effects are diminished, and often the person drinks more to achieve the desired effect. This increased dose can result in more desensitization and even higher doses. This begins the cycle of addiction.

Tolerance can vary between people with the same alcohol experience, as well as between different effects of alcohol in the same person. For example, a person may become tolerant to the cognitive effects of alcohol and not feel "drunk" while their physical effects (slowed reaction times, loss of balance, etc.) are still impaired. This can lead a person to drink more to achieve the desired cognitive effect, enhancing the negative physical effects, and to misjudge his or her ability to perform physical activities (driving, biking, skateboarding, etc.). The degree of tolerance developed varies from moderate users, who experience mild tolerance, to chronic, high-dose alcohol users who have extreme tolerance. It is not uncommon for chronic alcoholics to be arrested for driving under the influence with a BAC that would produce stupor or death in an infrequent alcohol user.

A number of different types of tolerance to alcohol have been categorized (see Table 7.1). *Acute tolerance* is a central effect that develops during a single session with alcohol and can begin within minutes of alcohol exposure. In acute tolerance, the subjective and behavioral effects are greater during the rise of alcohol in the blood than later when the BAC is at the same level or even greater. Thus, there is not a direct correspondence between BAC and the cognitive and behavioral effects of alcohol over time during a single event. Studies suggest that acute tolerance is mediated by phosphorylation of GABA and glutamate receptors. Phosphorylation decreases the sensitivity of the channels to alcohol and is quickly reversed when alcohol is absent.

A type of tolerance that is developed outside the CNS is *metabolic tolerance*. Here the exposure to alcohol causes an upregulation of the liver enzymes for the metabolism of alcohol, especially ADH and enzymes of the cytochrome P450

Table 7.1 Types of Tolerance

Type	Effect	Mechanism
Acute	Adaptation while drinking alcohol	Phosphorylation of GABA and glutamate receptors
Metabolic	Accelerated breakdown of alcohol	Upregulation of ADH and cytochrome P450
Pharmacologic	Decreased neuronal effect of alcohol	Downregulation of GABA and glutamate receptors
Learned	Psychological adaptation to alcohol	Learned mechanisms of hiding behavioral effects

group. This increases the first-pass effect and the amount of alcohol in the blood that is metabolized per hour. This causes both a decrease in the peak BAC for a given amount of alcohol ingested and an increase in the rate of alcohol removal from the blood. Paradoxically, metabolic tolerance reverses as chronic alcohol use damages the liver, which then becomes less able to metabolize the drug.

The direct effect of alcohol in the brain is diminished by a third type of tolerance, *pharmacological tolerance*. Chronic overstimulation of GABA receptors due to alcohol causes the cells expressing these receptors to downregulate them (see Receptor Regulation, Chapter 3). Conversely, blockage of glutamate receptors by alcohol causes cells to upregulate these receptors. The result of this is twofold. First, alcohol becomes less potent in the individual, and a higher dose must be taken to produce the same effect. Second, abrupt withdrawal of alcohol leaves the brain with too few GABA receptors and too many glutamate receptors. This causes hyperstimulation of the brain, leading to the dangerous withdrawal symptoms described below. Metabolic and neuronal tolerances are both forms of chronic tolerance, due to repeated exposure to alcohol. The extent of these types of tolerance is dependent on the length of time and the amount of alcohol used.

A final form of tolerance is *learned tolerance*. Learned tolerance involves a person learning to behave more normally while under the influence of alcohol. A person can learn to behave in ways to compensate for the cognitive effects of alcohol, and alcoholics often do this to hide their drinking. However, some effects of alcohol, such as the decrease in reaction time and uncoordinated movement, cannot be compensated for and make complicated tasks (e.g., driving) more dangerous.

Dependence and Withdrawal

Dependence occurs as the body adapts to the presence of alcohol. Dependence is due to the tolerance mechanisms described above that help the body adapt to living with alcohol. Once the body is in this altered state, the sudden removal of alcohol results in a lowered emotional set point (see Figure 5.8), which is felt as *withdrawal*. The body must revert back to its initial physiological state to feel normal in the absence of alcohol again, which takes time. Withdrawal can be divided into effects caused by acute and chronic use.

Some of the symptoms of acute alcohol bingeing (i.e., the hangover) are due to the neurological adaptation mechanisms discussed above as pharmacological tolerance. Changes in the phosphorylation and numbers of GABA and glutamate receptors can produce a hyperexcitable state in the CNS. Thus, while binge drinking may cause a person to sleep late afterward, the quality of sleep is poor due to this rebound hyperexcitability. Irritability and anxiety the following day are a result of these changes; this is why the age-old treatment for a hangover is a "hair of the dog that bit you." A low dose of alcohol on the following day can help alleviate the hyperexcitability.

Other symptoms of a hangover include increased heart rate and high blood pressure, headache, nausea and vomiting, thirst, fatigue, and depression. Some of these effects can be explained by the dehydration that accompanies alcohol abuse. The diuresis caused by the inhibition of antidiuretic hormone release (see above) causes blood pressure to drop, which results in a rebound increase in heart rate and blood pressure, resulting in headache and an overall feeling of fatigue. In addition, acute toxicity can contribute to the hangover. Acetaldehyde from alcohol metabolism is quite toxic, as are some side products of fermentation and distillation

Liver Disease

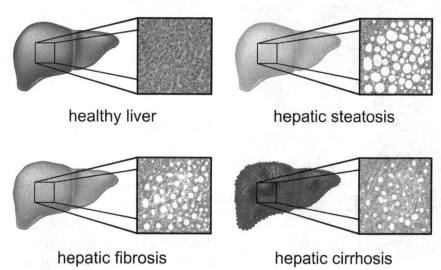

healthy liver

hepatic steatosis

hepatic fibrosis

hepatic cirrhosis

Figure 7.11 The first stage of liver damage involves storage of triglycerides in vacuoles of liver cells. This is called hepatic steatosis or fatty liver. Chronic storage of fat can lead to inflammation and cell death. Necrotic liver cells leave behind fibrous scar tissue, referred to as hepatic fibrosis. As this process proceeds, cells die and are replaced by scar tissue. The final stage of this is hepatic cirrhosis.

found in cheap liquors (e.g., methanol). These compounds produce inflammation, which causes headache, nausea, and vomiting.

Withdrawal symptoms from chronic abuse are much more severe and associated with the pharmacological tolerance. The chronic down-regulation of GABA receptors and upregulation of glutamate receptors make the person dependent on alcohol to avoid hyperexcitability. If alcohol is suddenly withdrawn, the brain becomes wildly overstimulated, resulting in tremors, sweating, heart palpitations, and visual and auditory hallucinations. The syndrome is called delirium tremens and can last two to four days after cessation of alcohol use. In extreme cases, this hyperexcitability can result in seizures and death. Chronic alcoholics are often treated with benzodiazepines, which activate GABA receptors, in order to taper them off alcohol while avoiding seizures.

Chronic Health Effects

Chronic alcohol abuse produces serious negative effects on the body. The most common is liver damage. The first stage, which can be induced by several days of heavy drinking, is a fatty liver (see Figure 7.11). Acetate made from the metabolism of alcohol in the liver is converted to fatty acids that are then conjugated into triglycerides and stored in large vacuoles inside the liver cells. This stresses the cells and, if it becomes a chronic problem, causes inflammation and cell death. At this stage, the liver is able to heal itself. However, if alcoholism progresses, the person may develop alcoholic hepatitis. During the inflammatory process of hepatitis, cells die and are replaced by fibrous material. This scarring of the liver can progress to cirrhosis of the liver. In cirrhosis, liver function has decreased significantly because most of the cells have died and have been

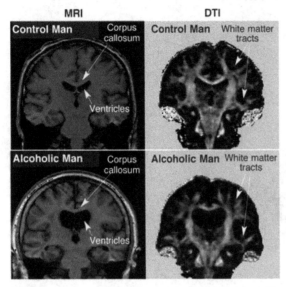

Figure 7.12 Chronic alcoholism and its related vitamin B1 deficiency causes dramatic brain shrinkage. Not the expanded size of the fluid-filled ventricles as well as the fissures in the cerebral cortex.

replaced with fibrous scar material. Cirrhosis of the liver accounts for 75% of all deaths due to alcoholism.

Brain damage is also common in chronic alcoholism, due to the toxic effects of chronically elevated alcohol and acetaldehyde in the brain. Vitamin B1 deficiency is another source of brain damage. Deficiency of water-soluble vitamins such as B1 is related to diuresis as well as poor nutrition that is common in alcoholics. This is called Wernicke–Korsakoff syndrome and can progress to Korsakoff's psychosis in its extreme form (see Figure 7.12). Liver dysfunction also contributes to this, as the liver is no longer able to process toxins that build up in the blood. Chronic alcoholism can cause the brain to shrink up to 25%, with concomitant changes in personality (confusion, agitation, anxiety) and loss of function (poor motor function, decreased reaction time, tremors).

The gastrointestinal tract is heavily damaged by chronic alcoholism. Gastritis and pancreatitis are common, especially when distilled spirits are consumed. Alcohol also promotes cancers, especially of the mouth, esophagus, and stomach.

Summary

Alcohol is the second most widely used recreational drug in the world. It is made by the anaerobic fermentation of any sugar-containing solution by yeast and bacteria. There are many forms of alcoholic beverages, varying in taste as well as concentration of alcohol. Alcohol is unique among drugs in that it is removed from the body at a constant rate, one drink per hour, by the enzyme alcohol dehydrogenase. The effects of alcohol are dose dependent, ranging from a mild relaxation (BAC 0.01 to 0.05%), to a loss of inhibitions and decreased reaction times (BAC 0.05 to 0.20%), to vomiting, stupor, and even death (BAC > 0.20%). Low-dose effects of alcohol are caused by a potentiation of GABA receptors and inhibition of glutamate receptors. This causes relaxation and an indirect release of dopamine in the limbic system, which produces both a pleasurable effect and an addiction potential. At high doses, alcohol acts like a general anesthetic, dissolving in the membranes of nerve cells, disrupting their function. Tolerance to the effects of alcohol builds due to several different mechanisms. Moderate daily intake of alcohol can have positive cardiovascular effects; however, chronic, high-dose use (alcoholism) leads to the destruction of the liver (cirrhosis) and brain shrinkage. Overuse of alcohol during pregnancy is strongly correlated with birth defects (fetal alcohol syndrome).

Further Reading

Alcohol and driving: Martin, T. L., P. A. Solbeck, D. J. Mayers, R. M. Langille, Y. Buczek, and M. R. Pelletier. "A Review of Alcohol-Impaired Driving: The Role of Blood Alcohol Concentration and Complexity of the Driving Task." *Journal of Forensic Sciences* 58 (2013): 1238–50.

Cardiovascular protection by alcohol: Chiva-Blanch G., S. Arranz, R. M. Lamuela-Raventos, and R. Ramon Estruch. "Effects of Wine, Alcohol and Polyphenols on Cardiovascular Disease Risk Factors: Evidences from Human Studies." *Alcohol and Alcoholism* 48 (2013): 270–7.

Alcohol and tolerance: Pietrzykowski, A. Z., and S. N. Treistman. "The Molecular Basis of Tolerance." *Alcohol Research & Health* 31 (2008): 298–309.

Alcohol withdrawal: Monte, R., R. Rabuñal, E. Casariego, H. López-Agreda, A. Mateos, and S. Pértega. "Analysis of the Factors Determining Survival of Alcoholic Withdrawal Syndrome Patients in a General Hospital." *Alcohol and Alcoholism* 45 (2010): 151–8.

Fetal alcohol spectrum disorder: Bakoyiannis, I., E. Gkioka, V. Pergialiotis, I. Mastroleon, A. Prodromidou, G. D. Vlachos, and D. Perrea. "Fetal Alcohol Spectrum Disorders and Cognitive Functions of Young Children." *Reviews in the Neurosciences* 25 (2014): 631–9.

Test Your Understanding
Multiple-Choice

1. Ethyl alcohol has _____ carbon(s), while methyl alcohol has _____ carbon(s).
   a. one, two
   b. one, three
   c. two, three
   d. two, one

2. Alcohol is first metabolized into
   a. acetaldehyde
   b. isopropanol
   c. acetic acid
   d. methanol

3. The low-dose effects of alcohol involve
   a. inhibiting GABA receptors
   b. inhibiting serotonin receptors
   c. inhibiting dopamine receptors
   d. inhibiting glutamate receptors

4. Alcohol causes dehydration because of
   a. inhibition of ADH release
   b. indirect release of endorphins
   c. nonspecific effects from dissolving in membranes
   d. indirect release of dopamine in the limbic system

5. The loss of inhibitions produced by alcohol is because of effects in the
   a. prefrontal cortex
   b. nucleus accumbens
   c. dorsal striatum
   d. cerebellum

6. Uncoordinated movements and speech produced by alcohol are due to effects in the
   a. prefrontal cortex
   b. nucleus accumbens
   c. dorsal striatum
   d. cerebellum

7. A type of tolerance that produces hyperexcitability in withdrawal is
    a. metabolic tolerance
    b. pharmacological tolerance
    c. learned tolerance
    d. all of the above
8. A 140-pound man would cross the threshold for legal intoxication if he drank ____ drinks in one hour.
    a. 2
    b. 3
    c. 4
    d. 5

Essay Questions

1. Describe four things that can affect BAC for a given amount of alcohol drunk.
2. What is the mechanism of action of low-dose alcohol? What is the mechanism of high-dose alcohol?
3. Alcohol is often called a "social lubricant." Why is this?
4. In the movie *Indiana Jones and the Raiders of the Lost Ark,* there is a scene where the female lead, Marion, trades shots with an older, larger man in her bar in Nepal. For every shot he takes, she takes one. Eventually he passes out, and she gets up and cleans up the bar. Give three reasons why this would be unlikely in real life. Also, how could this be possible in real life?
5. What is cirrhosis of the liver? Describe the process that leads to it.

Credits

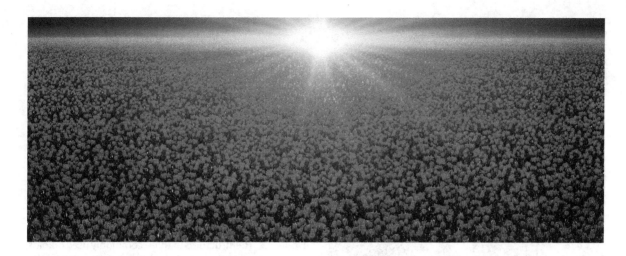

Chapter 8: Opioids

Introduction

Opioids are a class of drug called *analgesics*, which means "not feel pain." One major role of endogenous opioids, the peptide neurotransmitters endorphin and enkephalin, is to modulate the sensation of pain as it is sent from the body to the cerebral cortex, where it is perceived. The main reason opioid drugs are prescribed is to decrease pain sensation, for example, after surgery. There are other drugs that also modulate pain, for example, nonsteroidal anti-inflammatory drugs (NSAIDs: aspirin, ibuprofen, naproxen, and acetaminophen) and cannabinoids, but opioids are in their own class because they have specific receptors that they activate.

If the only effect of opioid drugs was to block pain, they would not be used recreationally (as NSAIDs are not) and would not be subject to abuse. In addition to pain modulation, endogenous opioids are important in the limbic system as part of the reward mechanism (see Chapter 5). On top of pain relief, opioids produce euphoria and a pleasant, dreamy state similar to but much stronger than the afterglow that follows orgasm. Thus, opioids are highly sought after for recreational use, and chronic recreational users of opioids are prone to addiction. Opioids also cause constipation, and specific opioids are used clinically for this effect. A major danger of opioid use is respiratory depression, and this is the main cause of death in overdose.

Opiates and Opioids

This class of drugs is very ancient in origin. Derived from the flower of the opium poppy, its botanical name, *Papaver somniferum*, means "poppy that brings sleep." It has been used by man since prehistorical times and has been continually cultivated since then.

Agonists

The herbal product derived from the poppy is opium. This is collected by slashing the unripe seed pod of the flower and collecting the juice that seeps out (see Figure 8.1). This produces a thick paste that can be eaten or smoked. Another common preparation is alcoholic extraction

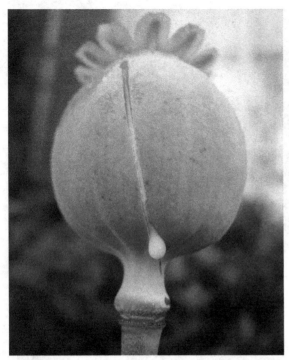

Figure 8.1 This is an unripe seedpod from the opium poppy. The pod exudes a sticky resin that is collected and dried to produce opium paste.

A

Morphine

B

Heroin

C

Fentanyl

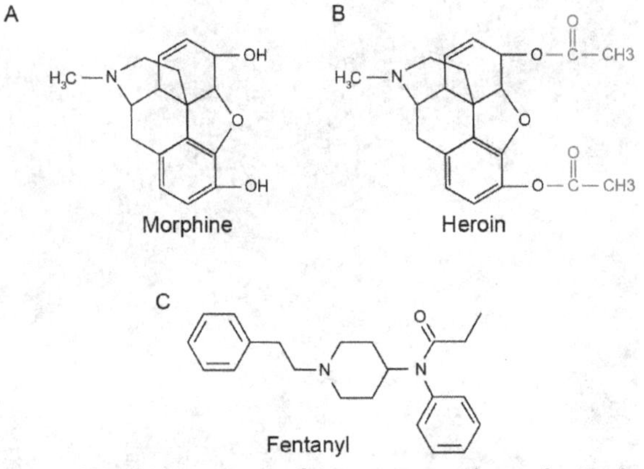

Figure 8.2 The structures of three commonly used opioids are shown. Note that heroin differs from morphine by the addition of two acetate groups. Fentanyl is a synthetic opioid and bears little similarity to morphine.

(tincture) of the opium. Products produced this way, called laudanum and paregoric, were commonly available until the early twentieth century. Opium contains a mixture of phytochemicals including several active compounds; the main active compounds in opium are morphine and codeine. These opiates were isolated from opium in the nineteenth century and are still commonly used medicinally.

The basic chemical structure of the natural opiates has been modified to make semisynthetic opioids (see Figure 8.2). The most commonly used examples are oxycodone (Percodan, OxyContin), hydrocodone (Vicodin), hydromorphone (Dilaudid), and diacetylmorphine (heroin). There are also entirely synthetic compounds called opioids (which bear no structural similarity to natural opiates) that activate the same receptors as the opiates. These include meperidine (Demerol), fentanyl (Sublimaze), and methadone (Dolophine). Over time, the distinction between opiates and opioids has become less important, and all drugs in this general class are typically referred to as opioids, irrespective of their origin.

Antagonists

In addition to these full agonists of the opioid receptors, there are partial agonists and antagonists. Buprenorphine is a partial agonist at these receptors. This means that it binds to the opiate receptors and activates them, but not fully. It is often used in addiction rehabilitation and will be discussed below. Antagonists of opioid receptors include naloxone (Narcan) and nalorphine (Nalline). These are used to reverse the life-threatening respiratory depression caused by opioid overdose.

Endogenous Agonists

As with many drugs, the opioids produce their effects by mimicking endogenous ligands. The endogenous opioids mimicked by these drugs are a group of peptide neurotransmitters called endorphins and enkephalins. Another endogenous opioid, dynorphin, produces effects that oppose the effects of endorphins and enkephalins.

Effects

The main effect of opioids, at low doses, is to decrease the perception of pain. At higher doses, they produce euphoria (called a "rush"), then a pleasant, dreamy state likened to the relaxed, happy feeling after orgasm. This is less euphoric and is more an overall sense of well-being ("everything is OK"). At high enough doses they produce sleep, which is why they are called narcotics. Other centrally produced effects are nausea, vomiting, and constricted pupils. Peripherally, opioids produce constipation by blocking gastrointestinal motility. Opioids depress breathing, which can cause death in overdose, as can aspiration of vomit produced by nausea.

Pharmacokinetics
Absorption and Distribution

The differences between different opioid agonists are mainly due to their pharmacokinetics, which are a result of their polarity metabolism. The uses and abuses of the opioids are determined by these parameters. Rather than list the details of all of the opioids (there are dozens), four representative agonists will be discussed: morphine, heroin, fentanyl, and methadone. The pharmacokinetics of each will be compared and contrasted. Each of these drugs can be taken orally, injected, snorted, or absorbed topically, which affects their rates of absorption. The intravenous route of administration is mainly discussed below.

Morphine is a somewhat polar drug (see Figure 8.2A). It is a weak base that is about 85% ionized at the body's pH, which means that only 15% of it can cross the blood-brain barrier at any one time (see Figure 8.3). As morphine moves into the brain, more in the blood becomes unionized and moves into the brain. This produces a slow, two-compartment distribution of the drug (see Figure 1.10). Even after IV administration, the time to peak in the brain is slow, about fifteen to thirty minutes. This gives morphine a

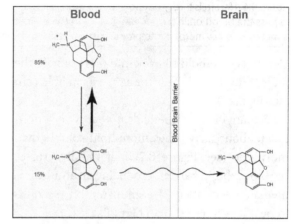

Figure 8.3 Two compartment model of morphine distribution. Morphine is an ionizable drug that is 85% ionized at the pH of the blood. Only the unionized form of morphine can cross the blood brain barrier. This slows the entry of morphine into the brain results in a two compartment model of distribution.

longer duration of action than other opioid drugs and makes it less addictive, making it clinically useful.

Heroin, on the other hand, is nonpolar. It is made by chemical treatment of opium paste to add two acetate groups to morphine's structure (thus, it is called diacetylmorphine). This blocks two polar hydroxyl groups (see Figure 8.2B) and helps heroin to get into the brain much faster than morphine, peaking approximately one minute after IV administration. These acetate groups pharmacologically inactivate the molecule.

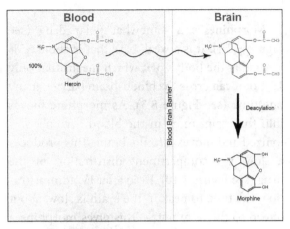

Figure 8.4 Heroin is a very nonpolar drug, which allows it to pass the blood brain barrier easily. Once in the brain it is metabolized to morphine to produce its effects.

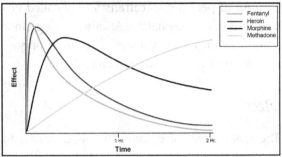

Figure 8.5 The different times to peak and durations of action of the drugs are important determinants of each drug's uses and abuse potential. Fentanyl is very nonpolar and peaks in the brain very quickly, diminishing rapidly over time. Morphine takes much longer to peak but stays at an effective dose longer. Heroin's pharmacokinetic profile is between these two, but closer to fentanyl than morphine. Methadone has a very slow absorption and peaks very slowly.

Heroin is metabolized back into morphine in the brain; thus, morphine is the active form of heroin (see Figure 8.4).

Fentanyl is a synthetic drug that is very nonpolar, about forty times more lipid soluble than morphine (see Figure 8.2C). It rapidly crosses the blood-brain barrier, producing an almost immediate effect after IV administration (seconds to peak), even faster than heroin.

As with most nonpolar drugs, the initial strong effect of a single large dose of heroin or fentanyl rapidly decreases (see Figure 8.5). This is because the drug initially partitions into the brain from the blood, resulting in a high brain concentration and a strong effect. Later, the concentration of the drug in the blood will decrease as it distributes into other fatty compartments in the body. The drug in the brain will then leach out into the blood and be redistributed to these compartments, diminishing its effect.

The different times to peak and durations of action of the drugs are very important determinants of their uses and abuse potential. A very rapid peak time of fentanyl is important for surgical applications. An anesthesiologist can rapidly induce analgesia and titrate to effect; that is, the amount of fentanyl needed to maintain anesthesia

is added as the patient is monitored. After surgery, the fentanyl is discontinued, and the anesthesia reverses quickly due to redistribution. The patient will awaken in thirty minutes but still feel groggy for hours later, as the drug is metabolized by the liver and eliminated. However, the rapid peak of fentanyl has a profound effect on its addictive potential. Drugs that peak quickly cause euphoria that builds faster than the anti-reward mechanism of the limbic system can counter it (see Figure 8.6). This produce a "rush" that makes them more

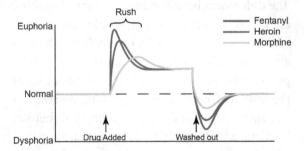

Figure 8.6 The polarity of the drug affects the time to peak; fentanyl is the fastest and morphine the slowest. This also affects the addictiveness of the drug because opioids that peak faster also peak higher and produce a greater rush. This rush is produced by dopamine release in the NA is and what is being sought by the users.

addictive. Heroin peaks quickly as well, although fentanyl is even more addictive because it peaks faster than heroin. Morphine, on the other hand, peaks much more slowly. As such, it is less addictive and much more commonly used clinically for pain management than anesthesia is.

Metabolism and Elimination

Opioid drugs, in general, are metabolized by the cytochrome P450 complexes in the liver. This means that they have a significant first-pass effect. This also means that the dose that reaches the bloodstream and the duration of effect can be highly variable. People can vary greatly in levels of P450 enzymes, both genetically and due to exposure to other drugs that affect cytochrome P450 expression. Opioids are metabolized to inactive, polar compounds by the cytochrome P450 enzymes, which are then excreted by the kidneys. Morphine, being rather polar to begin with, is partially excreted unchanged by the kidneys.

Chronic Pain Management

One drug that is an exception to the kinetics above is methadone. Methadone has a very slow onset of effect and long duration (see Figure 8.5). There are two main uses for methadone. It can be used for long-term management of chronic pain. The long duration of action eliminates the need for multiple daily dosing to manage pain. A more common use of methadone is for maintenance of addicts in recovery from addiction. This will be discussed more below.

Opioid agonists prescribed orally for pain management last approximately four hours and require repeat dosing for pain relief. This can be a difficult schedule to maintain for people dealing with chronic pain, for example, with cancer or arthritis. In 1995 the FDA approved a new product,

OxyContin, which is a controlled-release formulation of oxycodone (previously released as Percodan). OxyContin is compounded so that the oxycodone is released slowly from the pill as it passes through the digestive tract. The dose of oxycodone can be three to four times higher than Percodan. However, because it is released slowly, the peak concentration in the blood is comparable to Percodan, but maintained relatively constant for twelve hours instead of peaking and diminishing in four.

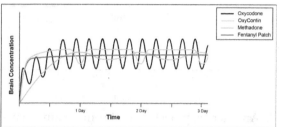

Figure 8.7 Multiple dosing with oxycodone produces a steady-state level after several administrations, with peaks and troughs related to the dosing interval. Controlled release oxycodone (OxyContin) increases the dosing interval and decreases the peaks and troughs. Methadone has a slow on and off rate and a steady-state level with minor peaks and troughs. Controlled release of fentanyl from a patch produces a steady-state level without peaks and troughs.

While this strategy was a boon to people with chronic pain, drug abusers quickly learned that the controlled-release intent of the medicine could be defeated by crushing the capsules into a powder. The powder can be then snorted, dissolved in water and injected, or swallowed. This provides immediate release of the oxycodone at a much higher dose than intended. OxyContin abuse proliferated as a result. In 2010, OxyContin was reformulated to reduce its addiction potential. The newer pills are harder to crush and do not break down into a powder or dissolve in water. As a result, many OxyContin abusers switched to heroin, which is cheaper and unregulated.

Table 8.1 Receptors, Endogenous Agonists, Locations, and Effects (by Location)

Receptor	Endogenous Agonist	Locations	Effects
μ-opioid (MOR)	Endorphin	NA VTA Thalamus RAS Raphe nucleus Medulla PAG Dorsal horn	Euphoria Euphoria Pain modulation Relaxation Well-being Respiratory depression Pain modulation Pain modulation
δ-opioid (DOR)	Enkephalin	NA Amygdala	Slight euphoria Relaxation
κ-opioid (KOR)	Dynorphin	NA Thalamus RAS Raphe nucleus	Dysphoria Pain modulation Anxiety Depression

Another approach to chronic pain management is the fentanyl transdermal patch (Duragesic). Transdermal patches are a method of delivering a constant supply of a nonpolar drug through a controlled-release skin patch (see Figure 1.8 and Figure 8.7). Fentanyl patches are prescribed for moderate to severe chronic pain. They are commonly abused by attaching more than prescribed or by changing the patch more frequently than recommended. Also, the physical barrier of the patch is easily torn open, releasing an alcoholic solution of the drug. This is snorted, smoked, or applied to the gums or other mucus membranes. This produces a fast, short-lived rush that is very addictive.

Receptors and Endogenous Agonists

Three Main Receptors

There are three main receptors for the endogenous opioids: mu (μ) opioid receptors (MORs), delta (δ) opioid receptors (DORs), and kappa (κ) opioid receptors (KORs). These receptors differ in location and which endogenous opioids are more selective for them (see Table 8.1). They are seven-transmembrane metabotropic receptors that interact with G-proteins (see Figure 3.8). Opioid receptors are inhibitory and act by a number of mechanisms.

MORs are found in all parts of the brain but are especially concentrated in the cortex, thalamus, nucleus accumbens (NA), ventral tegmental area (VTA), reticular activating system (RAS), raphe nucleus, and medulla, and on the axon bulbs of nociceptive neurons in the dorsal root ganglia. Endorphins have the highest affinity for the MORs, and opioids used for analgesia are primarily MOR agonists. Activation of MORs produces analgesia as well as euphoria, relaxation, and a profound sense of well-being through receptors in the VTA/NA, RAS, and raphe nucleus. Because they are linked to the VTA/NA reward pathway, these receptors are responsible for the addictive potential of opioid drugs. MORs in the thalamus are involved in the transmission of pain messages from the body to the cerebral cortex. MORs in

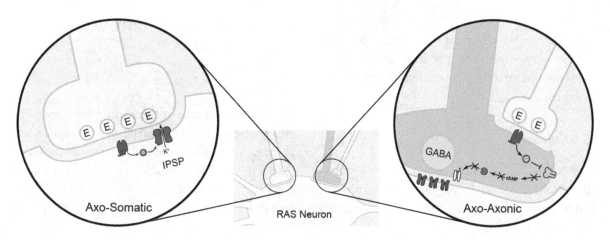

Figure 8.8 Opioid receptors can be found in axosomatic/dendritic synapses or axoaxonic synapses (center). In axosomatic/dendritic synapses (left), the receptors activate a G-protein that opens K⁺ channels. This produces an IPSP. In axoaxonic synapses (right), the receptors activate a G-protein that inhibits the production of cAMP by adenylyl cyclase (in green). This decreases cAMP the axon bulb, decreasing protein kinase A activation (PKA, in red). This leads to less phosphorylation of voltage dependent calcium channels (VDCCs, in yellow), less Ca²⁺ entry during an action potential, and less release of neurotransmitter (GABA).

the medulla are linked to respiration; activation of the MORs here slows respiration and can stop breathing in overdose.

DORs have a similar distribution to MORs, but are less dense. DORs are highly expressed in the olfactory bulb, as opposed to MORs, which are not. The endogenous agonists of the DORs are the enkephalins, and their effect on DORs is similar to that of endorphins on the MORs, but less so. Opioids that have been synthesized specifically for the DORs produce analgesia, but there is a ceiling to the effect; MOR agonists are more efficacious in countering pain. However, DOR agonists are not linked to addiction.

KORs are the opposite of MORs and DORS. They are found in the cortex, NA, thalamus, RAS, and raphe nucleus. The endogenous agonists of these receptors are the dynorphins, which produce dysphoria and depression. KORs are part of the anti-reward system, discussed in Chapter 5 as a means of downregulating the euphoria produced by dopamine in the NA. This is mainly through receptors in the NA and raphe nucleus. Agonists for these receptors, such as the active ingredients

in the plant *Salvia divinorum*, produce hallucinations and will be addressed in Chapter 10.

Receptor Activation

MORs and DORs are usually found on cell bodies/dendrites of neurons or on the presynaptic axon bulbs of GABAergic neurons (i.e., GABA-releasing neurons). Activation of MORs and DORs can affect postsynaptic cells in two ways. Opioid receptors on neuronal dendrites (axodendritic) or cell bodies (axosomatic) are linked to a G-protein that opens K⁺ channels (see Figure 8.8, left inset). Opening these channels hyperpolarizes the membrane and decreases the excitability of the postsynaptic membrane (IPSP). Opioid receptors may also be on the axon bulb of another neuron (axoaxonic transmission). These are linked to a G-protein that inhibits cAMP production (see Figure 8.8, right inset). This causes a decrease in the cAMP concentration in the axon bulb, a decrease in active protein kinase A, and a decrease in the phosphorylation of the voltage-dependent calcium channel.

This decreases incoming Ca^{2+} and therefore GABA release. The effect is less GABA release from the presynaptic bulb, decreasing the inhibition produced by GABA.

Disinhibition

The activation of the opioid receptors causes disinhibition through axoaxonic transmission. GABAergic neurons are inhibitory, deceasing activity in neurons by increasing Cl^- entry and producing IPSPs (see Figure 3.7B). Opioids inhibit GABA release, effectively inhibiting the inhibitor. This is called disinhibition; it causes indirect stimulation in the neurons that the GABA neuron was inhibiting. In the NA, this causes an increase of dopamine release from neurons that originate in the VTA (see Figure 5.4 and Figure 8.9).

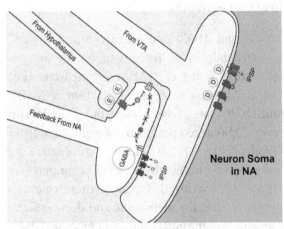

Figure 8.9 Feedback GABA-releasing axons from the NA make axoaxonic connections with dopamine releasing axon bulbs from the VTA. GABA receptors allow Cl^- entry, producing IPSPs that inhibit dopamine release. Endorphin-releasing axons from the hypothalamus make axoaxonic connections with the GABA axon bulbs. MORs in these synapses inhibit cAMP production, which results in less GABA release. In this way, endorphins are inhibiting the inhibitor (GABA), which is called disinhibition. (E = endorphin, D = dopamine)

Mechanisms of Action: One Drug, Two Effects
Painful Stimuli

As stated above, one of the main roles of endogenous opioids is to modulate the perception of pain. Pain is a very important stimulus in animals. It tells the individual that damage has been done (or is being done) to the body and action must be taken to minimize the damage. One type of response is a simple reflex arc, as in Figure 4.2, that quickly pulls the affected limb out of the way of the painful stimulus. These simple circuits don't include opioid receptors and are not subject to their effects. A more complicated pathway that is activated at the same time and by more prolonged painful stimuli includes axons that extend up the spinal cord to notify the CNS that there is serious damage. This pathway includes opioid receptors and is subject to modulation by opioid drugs.

Sensing pain is called nociception; the sensory neurons that perceive this are called nociceptive neurons. The cell bodies of these neurons are in the dorsal root ganglia (DRG; see Figure 8.7), neuron clusters alongside the spine. These are pseudo-unipolar neurons; they have a soma in the DRG and an axon that extends from the periphery (the distal process), bypasses the soma, and extends into the spine through the dorsal root (the proximal process). These are afferent neurons; they bring information into the central nervous system. Unlike interneurons, action potentials in sensory neurons are not produced by interactions with other neurons through synapses. Action potentials are generated by receptors at the end of the distal processes. Receptors here sense extremes in temperature, mechanical stress, and chemical exposure (e.g., chemicals produced during inflammation). Each nociceptive neuron is specific for one type of painful stimulus (e.g., cold vs. hot). Electrical shocks directly stimulate

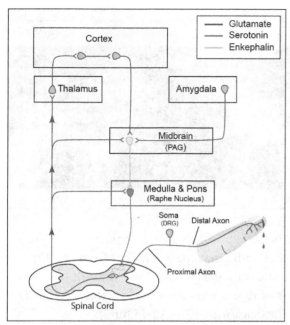

Figure 8.10 Painful stimuli are received by the distal axon of a neuron in the dorsal root ganglion (DRG). This is relayed through the dorsal root of the spinal cord by the proximal axon of this neuron. Interneurons in the spinal cord relay this to the hindbrain (medulla and pons), midbrain (periaqueductal gray matter, PAG), and thalamus. The thalamus relays this to the cortex. Feedback from the cortex and input from the amygdala stimulate cells in the PAG to release enkephalins in the raphe nucleus. The raphe nucleus releases serotonin in interneurons of the dorsal root of the spinal cord, which release enkephalins to inhibit pain transmission.

action potentials in sensory neurons and are very painful. These neurons are present in every peripheral part of the body (e.g., skin, joints, and internal organs) but are concentrated in some regions (e.g., hands and face).

The proximal axons from these nociceptive neurons enter the spine at the dorsal root and activate the interneurons of the simple reflexes (see Figure 4.2). They also stimulate neurons that project afferent axons to the CNS (see Figure 8.10). In the CNS, these axons simultaneously innervate neurons in the brain stem (medulla), midbrain (periaqueductal gray matter,

PAG), and thalamus. The thalamus relays this information to the cerebral cortex, which allows for the conscious perception of pain. The PAG receives input from the spinal neurons as well as feedback from the pain-receiving neurons in the cortex and the emotional centers in the limbic system (amygdala). The PAG modulates the pain pathway based on input from these higher centers. Descending (efferent) axons from the PAG interact with neurons in the medulla. These neurons project to the dorsal spinal cord, where the pain enters the CNS and releases endogenous opiates on the axon bulbs of the nociceptive neurons from the dorsal root (axoaxonic transmission). This decreases neurotransmitter release from the axon bulbs and, therefore, pain neurotransmission. This pathway is the source of the analgesia produced by opioid drugs, both centrally and in the spinal cord.

Euphoria, Relaxation, and Emotional Well-Being

Opioid receptors in the higher centers of the brain (cortex, limbic system, thalamus, RAS, and raphe nucleus) are important in both the emotional response to pain and in a person's stress response. This higher-order opioid mechanism produces a calming effect and distances the person from the pain.

As noted in Chapter 5, some of the feedback pathways in the limbic system that produce reward and anti-reward involve opioids (see Figure 5.5). GABAergic feedback neurons from the NA to the VTA, as well as GABAergic interneurons in the VTA and NA, inhibit release of dopamine in the limbic system (see Figure 8.10). Feedback from other areas of the limbic system (DS, cortex, amygdala) stimulates the NA-VTA inhibitory GABA connection via glutamate release. Endorphin-releasing neurons

Box 8.1: Opioids and Posttraumatic Stress Disorder

Posttraumatic stress disorder (PTSD) is a debilitating psychological condition (see Figure 8.12). The symptoms of PTSD include nightmares, insomnia, flashbacks, cue triggers, inability to talk about the events, depression, helplessness, hopelessness, and self-destructive behavior. PTSD is caused by prolonged, life-threatening stress, especially interpersonal stressors such as warfare,

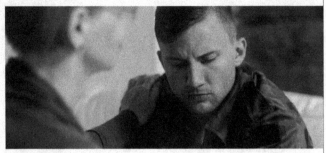

Figure 8.12

familial abuse, or sexual assault. In warfare, soldiers are exposed to an environment where they are chronically stressed and need to be hypervigilant. Death can come at any time from any direction. This is punctuated by episodes of extreme violence and the loss of close friends. It has been estimated that approximately 11 to 20% of veterans of recent wars show the symptoms of PTSD (https://medlineplus.gov/magazine/issues/winter09/articles/winter09pg10-14.html).

PTSD is usually the result of chronic rather than acute stress. Acute stress causes release of CRF in the VTA by the amygdala; this stimulates the VTA to release norepinephrine throughout the brain, causing hypervigilance. This effect is modulated by concurrent endorphin release. When the acute stress is relieved, CRF release abates and prolonged endorphin release helps the person relax. Chronic stress causes adaptive changes in this system. CRF receptors become downregulated, and endorphin release is increased. A new set point for stress has been established that helps the person survive this high-stress environment.

The downside of this adaptation is that soldiers become tolerant to the stress and dependent on endorphin release. The lack of stress when they return to safety is felt as opioid withdrawal, with classical withdrawal symptoms: anxiety and hypervigilance. This is caused by the decrease in chronic endorphin release when returning home, which allows more RAS stimulation and the release of norepinephrine. This increase in norepinephrine causes chronic anxiety. As a result, former soldiers tend to seek out dangerous, stressful situations (e.g., bar fights) or become addicted to drugs that stimulate MORs (alcohol and opioids).

from the hypothalamus modulate this GABA activity. They synapse with the GABA-releasing axon bulbs and inhibit GABA release (axoaxonic transmission). These receptors are mainly MORs. Activation of these receptors produces disinhibition of dopamine release in the limbic system, indirectly increasing stimulation of the reward pathway. In addition, there are MORs and DORs in the NA that directly produce euphoric reward, similar to dopamine, via K$^+$ channel activation. Stimulating these receptors, especially with opioid drugs, directly and indirectly produces the reward that leads to addiction.

Opioids also play a role in the response to stress (see Figure 8.11). Stress causes the release

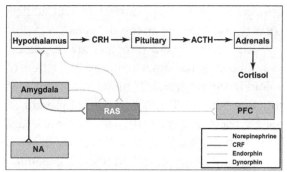

Figure 8.11 Stress messaging from the amygdala is initiated in two ways. CRF neurons from the amygdala stimulate the hypothalamus to release corticotropin-releasing hormone (CRH) to the pituitary. The pituitary responds by releasing adrenocorticotropic hormone (ACTH) into the blood; in the adrenal cortex, ACTH causes the release of cortisol. In the second pathway, CRF releasing axons from the amygdala stimulate the RAS to release norepinephrine in the prefrontal cortex and throughout the brain, producing anxiety and excitement. This is the stress pathway. The hypothalamus and amygdala inhibit the RAS by the release of endorphins. This is the anti-stress pathway.

of the neurotransmitter corticotropin-releasing factor (CRF), mentioned briefly in the discussion of the anti-reward pathway in Chapter 5. Neurons in the amygdala send CRF-releasing axons to synapse in the hypothalamus and the RAS. CRF stimulates the hypothalamus to cause the pituitary gland to release adrenocorticotropic hormone (ACTH). ACTH is carried by the bloodstream to the adrenal glands, which release cortisol in response. Cortisol is a major stress hormone in the body. This is called the hypothalamus-pituitary-adrenal (HPA) axis.

The CRF released in the RAS stimulates it to release norepinephrine throughout the brain and produce stimulation. Thus, the effect of CRF in the RAS is to produce an anxious, excited, hypervigilant state. This is the excited anxiety that accompanies acute fear produced by the amygdala. CRF produces this effect via metabotropic receptors that stimulate cAMP production and inhibit K^+ channel activation. This produces long-lasting

EPSPs in the norepinephrine-releasing neurons of the RAS.

In the same way that reward pathways activate anti-reward pathways, this anxiety-producing pathway also activates its opposite. Axons from the amygdala and hypothalamus synapse with these neurons in the RAS and release endorphins. These neurotransmitters activate MORs receptors, which do the opposite of CRF receptors; they inhibit the production of cAMP and activate K^+ channels (see Figure 8.8). This decreases action potential firing in the RAS, causing less norepinephrine to be released throughout the brain. The result is a calm, relaxed state. This helps relieve the stress induced by extreme fear or pain. The opioid pathway stays active for a while after the stress-inducing CRF pathway stops. This is why it feels good to be terrified by scary movies or amusement park rides; after the fear, you feel the relaxed, happy aftereffect of the endorphin release.

A third important CNS location of MORs is the raphe nucleus. These cells are also innervated by endorphin-releasing neurons from the hypothalamus and amygdala, similar to the RAS. Axons from the raphe nucleus extend down the spinal cord to the dorsal horn (see Figure 8.10). These neurons release enkephalins to diminish pain perception. Ascending axons from the raphe nucleus go through the medial forebrain bundle and release serotonin throughout the cerebral cortex. Activation of MORs in the raphe nucleus causes this release of serotonin. In the PFC, serotonin affects mood, producing a relaxed and confident feeling.

Together, the effects of opioids on the NA, RAS, and raphe nucleus produce a calm, relaxed, happy feeling. In the natural release of endorphins, this helps distance the person from the anxiety and fear that accompanies pain and also produces the relaxed, happy feeling after an orgasm. However, overstimulation of the MORs

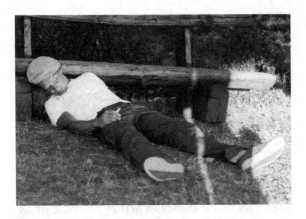

Figure 8.13 This picture shows an opioid abuser high on heroin.

by opioid abuse takes this to an extreme. It causes an extremely euphoric, relaxed, happy, dreamy state, likened to a whole-body orgasm that lasts for hours. This is called being "on the nod" (see Figure 8.13); it follows the rush that opioid abusers are seeking.

Negative Effects

In addition to the relaxed, happy feeling produced by CNS-MOR activation, these receptors in the medulla also cause respiratory depression. This is mild at low doses, progressing to profound depression and complete cessation at higher doses. In addition, opioid agonists stimulate the area postrema (chemical trigger zone) in the medulla, producing nausea and potentially vomiting. The combination of respiratory depression and vomiting/aspiration is a common cause of death in overdose. The respiratory depression can be quickly reversed with the use of an antagonist such as naloxone (Narcan). This competes for binding to the same receptors as opioids but keeps the receptors in the inactive state. This blocks the activity of the opioid agonists and converts the person immediately from overdose to full withdrawal.

Emergency room physicians report that addicts are very displeased when this happens.

Peripherally, opioid receptors are important in modulating intestinal motility. Activation of opioid receptors decreases motility, causing constipation in users. This is true both of prescribed opioid users and recreational abusers. Drugs have been developed to take advantage of these intestinal MORs to control diarrhea. Loperamide is a synthetic MOR agonist that is available over the counter for control of diarrhea. Loperamide has very little central effects because it doesn't appreciably cross the blood-brain barrier. On the other hand, people prescribed opioids have the unfortunate side effect of chronic constipation. They can find relief from opioid-induced constipation by using a newly released drug, naloxegol. This similar to loperamide in that it doesn't cross the blood-brain barrier; however, naloxegol is an antagonist at MORs. This allows for the central pain-relieving effects of opioids while blocking the peripheral side effects.

Tolerance, Dependence, and Treatment
Tolerance

Tolerance to opioids develops quickly at the receptor level as the MOR numbers and activity are downregulated. The receptors become less sensitive to agonists and less capable of activating G-proteins, and internalize due to phosphorylation (see Figure 3.11). This results in larger doses being needed to produce the desired high. This is sometimes called "chasing the dragon." Naive users may start by injecting 10 milligrams of heroin (or smoking 25 milligrams), while tolerant users will increase this as much as ten- to twentyfold, injecting more than a gram per day in multiple doses. This is particularly dangerous in that drugs bought on the street are not standardized for dose and may even be cut with other drugs (e.g., fentanyl) to increase their effect. Dose is particularly important because the safety ratio for heroin is approximately two- to threefold (see Figure 10.10). Doubling a dose can easily cause death. The variability in product, narrow range of safety, and need to increase the dose often lead to overdose.

Use will also typically graduate from snorting or smoking prescription opioids to injecting heroin. The bioavailability of opioids is much greater by injection, as the entire drug is put directly into the bloodstream. Smoking and snorting both require higher doses, which becomes cost prohibitive as tolerance increases. Injecting heroin becomes the least expensive alternative.

Dependence

As tolerance develops, so does dependence. The brain adapts to functioning in the presence of opioids and no longer functions well in their absence. This results in withdrawal during abstinence. Chronic overstimulation by opioids causes dopamine receptors in the NA to become downregulated, and stores of dopamine in the VTA become depleted. Anti-reward pathways, which produce dysphoria, are upregulated. These changes alter the set point for feeling normal. The addict no longer feels comfortable in the absence of opioids, must take them to feel normal, and doesn't get as high from taking them (see Figure 5.9). Prefrontal cortex activity switches from normal goal-directed activities to exclusive drug-seeking behavior (drug craving), as normal daily activities no longer provide pleasure. Upregulated connections from the DS to the NA cause compulsive drug seeking, which is difficult to inhibit by the normal PFC pathways that control behavior. Neurons of the RAS, which are chronically inhibited by abused opioids, become tonically more active. This decreases the effect of opioids and results in hyperactivity (nervous, anxious behavior) in their absence. The overall result is depression, insomnia, agitation, anxiety, muscle aches, chills/sweats, vomiting, diarrhea, and intense craving for the drug. The severity of the symptoms is affected by the length of time the person uses the drug, how much is used per day, and previous abstinence/withdrawals. The more times a person withdraws from the drugs, the more intense the withdrawal symptoms are.

Treatment

Chronic opioid abuse produces neuroadaptations that make sustained abstinence difficult. More than 90% of people who go through rehabilitation to stop using opioids relapse within a year. For this reason, treatment often involves maintenance with an opioid that is less behaviorally debilitating than opioids of abuse, methadone. Methadone has a slow absorption (when given orally) and a long half-life (fifteen to sixty hours, with much variability between users due to differences in liver metabolism of the drug). The slow onset of methadone effects eliminates the rush and deceases the narcotic effect that makes functioning difficult. The long half-life means that it can be taken once or twice daily to help the addict avoid withdrawal. This slow profile levels out the peaks and troughs caused by multiple dosing of fast-acting opioids (see Figure 8.5). Methadone doesn't cure the addiction, but maintains recovering addicts in a state where they can function.

Another drug used for opioid addiction is buprenorphine. Buprenorphine is a partial agonist at MORs, activating them only partially. This makes the danger of respiratory failure during overdose less likely. It also produces less downregulation of MORs than methadone does, which can aid in recovery. Suboxone is a mix of buprenorphine and naloxone intended to decrease rush, in case the user injects it rather than taking it orally as designed. Buprenorphine has shown promise for the treatment of addiction to other drugs as well, such as alcoholism, because other addictive drugs indirectly cause endorphin release. An exciting new treatment is buprenorphine implants called Probuphine; these are rods inserted under the skin to provide a continual release of buprenorphine over a six-month period. This has been effective in curbing withdrawal and cravings for this extended period.

Summary

Opioids are ancient drugs, having been used by humanity since prehistoric times. Natural, semisynthetic, and synthetic forms are available that vary in their pharmacokinetic profiles. Very nonpolar drugs, such as fentanyl, are useful clinically for their immediate pain-relieving and narcotic effects, but are more addictive. Less polar drugs, such as morphine, are also useful for pain relief and are less addictive because of their slow onset, especially when taken orally. There are three types of opioid receptors, MORs, DORs, and KORs. MORs and DORs are linked to analgesic, euphoric, and narcotic effects of opioids, while KORs produce dysphoria. Opioid receptors are found in many locations in the CNS and peripherally and therefore have many effects. The most important clinical effect is anti-nociception, or pain relief. This is due to receptors in the PAG and in interneurons of the dorsal root of the spinal cord. Opioids also produce euphoria and a calm, relaxing feeling. These effects are produced by receptors in the NA, RAS, and raphe nucleus. These are the effects sought by abusers of opioid drugs and are mainly produced by MORs. Chronic abuse of opioids causes a downregulation of the pathways that lead to these pleasant effects and an upregulation of anti-reward pathways. This causes withdrawal in abstinence and dependence on opioids. Sustained abstinence is difficult due to neuroadaptations that occur during abuse. Most treatment involves maintenance of the addict with opioid replacement drugs that decrease the highs and lows of chronic, daily abuse.

Further Reading

OxyContin abuse: Gudin, J. "Comparing the Effect of Tampering on the Oral Pharmacokinetic Profiles of Two Extended-Release Oxycodone Formulations with Abuse-Deterrent Properties." *Pain Medicine* 16 (2015): 2142–51.

Opioids and pain: Fields, H. "State-Dependent Opioid Control of Pain." *Nature Reviews Neuroscience* 5 (2004): 565–75.

Mood: Burgdorfa, J., and J. Pankseppa. "The Neurobiology of Positive Emotions." *Neuroscience & Biobehavioral Reviews* 30 (2006): 173–87.

Amygdala-RAS connection: Valentino, R. J., and E. Van Bockstaele. Endogenous Opioids: The Downside of Opposing Stress." *Neurobiology of Stress* 1 (2015): 23–32.

Treatment: Kosten, Thomas R., and Tony P. George. "The Neurobiology of Opioid Dependence: Implications for Treatment." *Science & Practice Perspectives* 1 (2002): 13–20.

Test Your Understanding

Multiple-Choice

1. Which of the following is an entirely synthetic opioid?
   a. morphine
   b. heroin
   c. fentanyl
   d. none of the above

2. Which of the following is the most nonpolar and addictive opioid?
   a. morphine
   b. heroin
   c. fentanyl
   d. none of the above

3. What is the opioid receptor for the endorphins?
   a. MOR
   b. DOR
   c. KOR
   d. dopamine receptor

4. When MORs are on the soma, they _____, and when they are on axon bulbs, they _____.
   a. open Na$^+$ channels, open Cl$^-$ channels
   b. open Cl$^-$ channels, inhibit cAMP production
   c. open K$^+$ channels, open Cl$^-$ channels
   d. open K$^+$ channels, inhibit cAMP production

5. What is the area in the midbrain that sends descending axons to modulate pain?
   a. VTA
   b. RAS
   c. raphe nucleus
   d. PAG

6. Which part of the brain sends both CRF and endorphin-releasing axons to the RAS?
   a. nucleus accumbens
   b. hypothalamus
   c. amygdala
   d. VTA

7. The overall sense of well-being produced by opioids is caused by the release of
   a. norepinephrine
   b. dopamine
   c. serotonin
   d. all of the above

8. The overdose potential of opiates is because of MORs in the
   a. medulla
   b. pons
   c. midbrain
   d. thalamus

Essay Questions

1. Discuss the chemical and pharmacological relationship between morphine and heroin.

2. Why is methadone used in the treatment of heroin addiction? Is this a cure?

3. The effect of MORs in the NA is called disinhibition. What is disinhibition, and what is the result of activating MORs?

4. In the movie *Pulp Fiction*, a female character snorts pure heroin, thinking that it is cocaine, and overdoses. In the next scene, a friend injects epinephrine directly into her heart, and she instantly revives. In actuality, epinephrine would not produce this result, but there is a drug that could. What is the drug, and how does it work?

5. The development of tolerance, which rapidly diminishes the effects of opioids, paradoxically results in an increase in overdose deaths. Why is this?

Credits

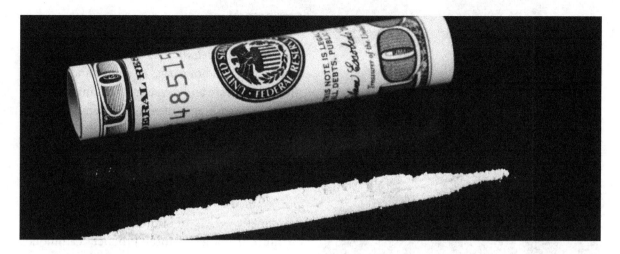

Chapter 9: CNS Stimulants

Introduction

The central nervous system (CNS) stimulants cocaine and amphetamine represent two drugs of very different structures with similar mechanisms of action and effects. Cocaine is a natural product, isolated from the coca plant, while amphetamine is synthesized from a natural product, ephedrine. Both of these drugs increase dopamine, norepinephrine, and serotonin in the brain, causing euphoria, stimulation, and self-confidence. Both are highly addictive.

While they are similar in many respects, there are important differences between them. Chief among the differences is the duration of action of the drugs; amphetamine is a much longer-acting drug than cocaine is. Also, there are major differences between the water-soluble forms of the drugs and their respective nonpolar, free-base forms that affect their addiction potential. Cocaine and amphetamines will be discussed separately, beginning with cocaine.

Cocaine

Cocaine is isolated from the leaves of the *Erythroxylon coca* plant (see Figure 9.1), which is native to South America. This nondescript bush, called the coca plant, has been cultivated for more than one thousand years by indigenous people of this area for use as a stimulant and appetite suppressant. The leaves are mixed with a basic substance (often ashes of quinoa stalks) and chewed to provide oral absorption of the cocaine through the mucous membranes. Cocaine is thought to be evolutionarily advantageous to the plant because of its insecticidal properties, although its relationship with man has been much more profitable to its long-term survival.

Cocaine was first isolated effectively from coca leaves in the mid-nineteenth century by Albert Nieman. Through the rest of the nineteenth century, it was available at pharmacies as an additive to drinks, especially alcoholic drinks, and as a powder. Injection of cocaine dissolved in water became popular as a local anesthetic and a treatment for depression and fatigue. Sigmund Freud was a strong proponent of the drug until he realized its addiction potential. The dangers of cocaine addiction became clear by the early twentieth century, at which time it was made illegal in the United States with the passage of the Harrison

Amphetamines

The name *amphetamine* is both the name of a specific drug and of a class of compounds with a similar structure and the same mechanism of action. Amphetamine is the original, semisynthetic drug of this class, having been synthesized from the natural compound ephedrine in 1887 (see Figures 9.2B and 9.2C). Ephedrine was isolated from the Chinese herb ma-huang (*Ephedra vulgaris*) and used for asthma (one of the sympathomimetic effects of stimulants is bronchiolar dilation). Another natural product, cathinone (see Figure 9.2E), derived from khat (or qat, *Catha edulis*), is structurally similar to ephedrine and also a stimulant used recreationally. Methamphetamine (see Figure 9.2D) is a compound that is synthesized from either ephedrine or pseudoephedrine (an optical diastereomer of ephedrine).

The effects of amphetamines are similar to that of cocaine except for the local anesthetic effect of cocaine, which is lacking in amphetamines. Amphetamines are both sympathomimetic and a CNS stimulant/euphoriant, with a mechanism of action similar to cocaine. The main difference is the longer duration of action of amphetamines.

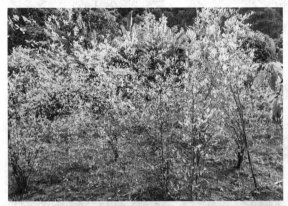

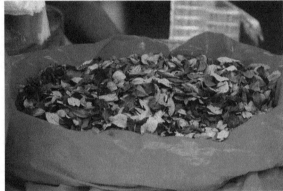

Figure 9.1

Narcotic Act in 1914. Cocaine then became scarce in the United States until the emergence of a drug culture in the late 1960s, and it has been a popular recreational drug since then.

There are three main effects of cocaine, based on two distinct mechanisms of action. Cocaine is a local anesthetic, blocking the transmission of action potentials in the axons of afferent sensory neurons. It is also a sympathomimetic, mimicking the sympathetic nervous system. In this role, it causes an increase in heart rate and vasoconstriction (which leads to high blood pressure) and relaxes airway passages. Finally, cocaine in the CNS produces euphoria, stimulation, and self-confidence. This is the effect that is sought out recreationally.

Pharmacokinetics of Cocaine
Absorption of Cocaine

As with other drugs, the absorption of cocaine is strongly affected by its structure and polarity. Cocaine is called an alkaloid because it has an amine as part of its structure, making it basic when dissolved in water. The nitrogen of the amine can be protonated or not, greatly changing its polarity. During its purification, coca paste is treated with hydrochloric acid (HCl) to make it

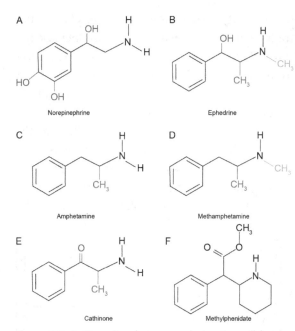

Figure 9.2 A. Norepinephrine; amphetamines all have a similar structure to norepinephrine with 2 OH groups (in blue) removed. B. Ephedrine, a natural product from ma huang that was used to synthesize amphetamine. C. & D. Amphetamine and methamphetamine; the two forms most often used recreationally. E. Cathinone; a natural product from khat. F. Methylphenidate; structurally very different from the others in this class.

and the crystals are recovered. This produces a purer form of freebase than crack (lacking the included water and bicarbonate), but it is very dangerous to produce because of the extreme flammability of ether.

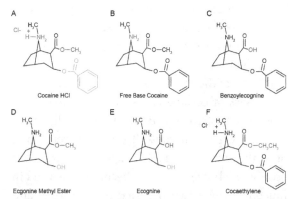

Figure 9.3 A. & B. Cocaine HCl and its free base. The ionizable amine group is in red. C., D., & E. The main inactive metabolites of cocaine. These are produced by hydrolysis of the methyl ester group (in blue, benzoylcognine), the benzoyl group (in green, ecogonine methyl ester) or both (ecognine). Benzoylcognine (C.) is the major product. F. Cocaethylene is formed in the blood by the combination of cocaine and ethanol. It has a longer half-life than cocaine.

water soluble. The acid protonates cocaine and adds the accompanying chloride anion, resulting in cocaine HCl (see Figure 9.3A, in red). This is the powder form of cocaine (see Figure 9.4A), which forms tiny crystals upon precipitation. Cocaine HCl can be treated with a base (usually sodium bicarbonate) and then dried. This removes the proton from the amine and makes it nonpolar (see Figure 9.3B). This nonpolar "freebase" form, called crack, produces larger crystals (see Figure 9.4A) that are somewhat opaque due to the inclusion of water. Freebase cocaine can also be made by dissolving cocaine HCL in water and precipitating it with ammonia, which converts it to the freebase form, making it insoluble in water. The freebase is then extracted from the water with ether, the ether is evaporated away,

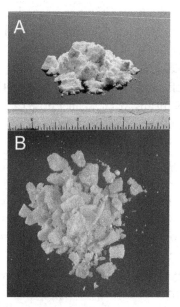

Figure 9.4

Differences in physical properties between cocaine HCl and freebase cocaine affect their use, sale, and addiction potential. Cocaine HCl breaks down in heat, so users take it by nasal insufflation (snorting) or by dissolving it in water and injecting it intravenously. Intravenous injection produces a faster peak (approximately three minutes) than insufflation does (approximately fifteen minutes), which increases the euphoric rush. It also ensures that 100% of the cocaine is absorbed, whereas only 30 to 60% of cocaine is absorbed when snorted. The vasoconstrictive activity of cocaine limits its nasal absorption because it decreases the blood flow through the nasal tissues. With repeated dosing, unabsorbed cocaine becomes dissolved in mucous, drips down the back of the throat, and is absorbed in the small intestine, where first-pass metabolism inactivates most of it. However, injection carries with it social and personal taboos, so cocaine HCl is usually snorted.

Crack cocaine is heat stable and can be smoked as well as snorted. It is typically not injected because it is not soluble in water. Smoking cocaine produces the fastest absorption, reaching the brain in seconds and peaking in ninety seconds. The rapid absorption produces the greatest rush and makes the drug extremely addictive. Approximately 70% of the cocaine is absorbed after inhalation, making it more efficient than snorting cocaine HCl. This efficiency means that a smaller dose can be taken, reducing the price per dose for crack.

Distribution of Cocaine

Whether cocaine is ingested as cocaine HCl or freebase cocaine, it becomes the freebase in the pH of the bloodstream and easily passes the blood-brain barrier. As with other nonpolar drugs, it partitions into the brain on its first pass via a two-compartment model (see Figure 1.10). It then slowly leaches out of the brain and is redistributed

to other fatty tissues. Slower methods of administration delay the time to peak but also increase the time that the drug is at an effective concentration in the brain (see Figure 9.5). Thus, the high from smoked crack cocaine lasts between five and fifteen minutes, while snorted cocaine HCl will last approximately forty-five minutes. In either method, but especially for smoked crack, the redistribution rapidly diminishes the high after its peak, causing the user to crave more and re-administer the drug. Cocaine is eventually transported to the liver to be metabolized.

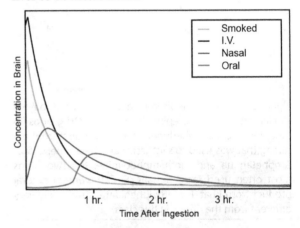

Figure 9.5 This represents the hypothetical time course of an equivalent dose of cocaine smoked, injected intravenously, snorted, and ingested orally. Both the time course of the effect and the peak concentration is affected by the route of administration.

Metabolism and Elimination of Cocaine

Cocaine has an easily hydrolyzed ester group (noted in blue in Figure 9.3A) that is rapidly removed by enzymes in the liver. This produces benzoylecgonine (see Figure 9.3C), the major metabolite (75%), which is polar and therefore excluded from the brain. The benzoyl ester (noted in green in Figure 9.3A) can also be hydrolyzed, producing ecgonine methyl ester (see Figure 9.3D), another polar metabolite. Cocaine has a short half-life in the blood, approximately fifty minutes. Benzoylecgonine and ecgonine methyl ester have much longer half-lives (approximately six and four hours, respectively) and are eliminated by the kidneys. Thus, cocaine use is detected via urinalysis for its metabolites. Because the metabolites can be detected at concentrations much lower than those needed for effect, they can be detected in urine up to a week after acute use and longer after chronic use, as the nonpolar cocaine slowly leaches out of fatty tissue, is metabolized, and is excreted.

The metabolism of cocaine is greatly affected by the concomitant use of alcohol. In the liver, the methyl ester of cocaine (in blue in Figure 9.3A) is exchanged for ethanol, producing the ethyl ester cocaethylene (see Figure 9.3F). Cocaethylene also crosses the blood-brain barrier and produces the same effects as cocaine. The main difference is that cocaethylene has a longer half-life (two hours), so co-use of alcohol with cocaine increases the duration of the effects.

Pharmacokinetics of Amphetamines

The drugs that are part of the amphetamine class are all structurally similar to the catecholamines norepinephrine and dopamine (see Figure 9.2). The major difference is the hydroxyl groups that define the catechol ring (in blue) are removed in amphetamines. This makes the drugs considerably less polar. Methylphenidate (Ritalin; see Figure 9.2F) is an exception to this rule, in that its structure is not similar to the catecholamine structure.

Absorption of Amphetamines

Amphetamine (see Figure 9.2C), marketed as either Benzedrine or Dexedrine, was designed as an orally administered stimulant, as was methylphenidate (see Figure 9.2F). Because these drugs are nonpolar, they can also be snorted and are often injected. Methamphetamine (see Figure 9.2D) is similar to cocaine in that it is available in both an HCl form and a freebase form. Methamphetamine HCL is a powder, often called crank or speed (see Figure 9.6A). It is destroyed by heat, so it is usually snorted or injected. Freebase methamphetamine is called by many names, including crystal meth, crystal, meth, glass, and ice. It is a crystallized form of methamphetamine that is heat stable and can be smoked, snorted, or dissolved and injected (see Figure 9.6B). Of these three drugs, methamphetamine is most often used recreationally because it is more available on the street (having been made in clandestine labs) than the pharmaceutically

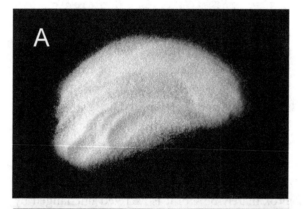

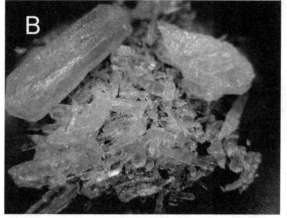

Figure 9.6

synthesized amphetamine and methylphenidate are.

Snorting, injecting, and inhaling methamphetamine are very rapid means of absorption. They produce a rapid high with a significant rush. Oral absorption produces a much slower onset, with less rush. Unlike cocaine, the method of absorption does not appreciably affect the duration of action of the methamphetamine because it has a very long half-life, although it does affect the addiction potential.

Distribution, Metabolism, and Elimination of Amphetamines

As with cocaine, the pH of the blood makes amphetamines nonpolar, and they easily pass through the blood-brain barrier. Unlike cocaine, the half-lives of amphetamines are very long. Both amphetamine and methamphetamine are poorly metabolized and have half-lives of approximately ten hours. They are removed from the blood very slowly, and therefore the drug in the brain forms an equilibrium with that in the blood. The stimulant effects of a methamphetamine high can last twelve to twenty-four hours.

Amphetamine is poorly metabolized; approximately 35% of it is excreted unchanged by the kidneys. Methamphetamine is metabolized to amphetamine as well as inactive chemicals. Approximately 40% of methamphetamine is excreted unchanged, and 10% is excreted as amphetamine. The rest is metabolized to inactive ingredients before excretion.

Figure 9.7 compares and contrasts the pharmacokinetics of the two different forms of cocaine and methamphetamine. The freebase forms of both drugs are usually smoked, while the HCl forms are usually snorted or injected. However they are taken, once they are in the body, the duration of action is dependent on the chemical itself; cocaine is short-acting, and methamphetamine is long-acting.

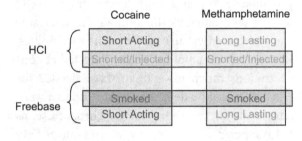

Figure 9.7

Mechanisms of Action of Cocaine and Amphetamines
Cocaine

There are three different physiological effects of cocaine, produced by two distinct mechanisms of action (see Table 9.1). A mechanism of action of cocaine that distinguishes it from amphetamines is that of a sodium channel blocker (see Figures 9.8A and 9.8B). This is the mechanism that makes it useful as a local anesthetic, using the same mechanism as lidocaine (Xylocaine) and procaine (Novocain). Blocking Na^+ channels stops action potential generation in nociceptive and other sensory neurons. This was one of the original uses for cocaine clinically, but it was replaced when other longer-acting Na^+ channel blockers became available. The local anesthetic effect isn't necessarily a recreational use, although users often rub residual cocaine on their gums after snorting and find the numbness produced to be pleasurable.

The second mechanism of action is in blocking the reuptake of the monoamine neurotransmitters dopamine, norepinephrine, and serotonin (see Figures 9.8C and 9.8D). It does this by binding to and inhibiting the presynaptic amine pump that removes the neurotransmitter from the synapse. This causes the neurotransmitter

Table 9.1 Acute and Chronic Effects of Cocaine and Amphetamines

Drug	Neurotransmitte	Mechanism	Acute Effect	Chronic Effect
Cocaine	None	Blocks voltage-dependent sodium channels	Local anesthetic	Cardiac arrhythmias
Cocaine, amphetamines	Norepinephrine, peripheral	Blocking/reversing NE reuptake pump	Sympathomimetic: increased heart rate, vasoconstriction, hypertension, bronchiolar dilation, glucose release, pupil dilation	Congestive heart failure, early onset dementia, peripheral necrosis
Cocaine, amphetamines	Norepinephrine, central	Blocking/reversing NE reuptake pump	Activation of RAS: excitement, energy, exhilaration	Toxic paranoid psychosis, ADHD, OCD
Cocaine, amphetamines	Dopamine, central	Blocking/reversing DA reuptake pump	Activation of limbic system: euphoria	Addiction, anhedonia
Cocaine, amphetamines	Serotonin, central	Blocking/reversing 5-HT reuptake pump	Activation of raphe nucleus: self-confidence, positive mood	Major depression

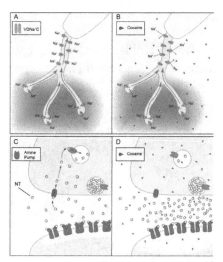

Figure 9.8 A. Stimulatory receptor channels (green) at the ends of nociceptive neurons sense painful stimuli (red) and relay this excitation (EPSPs) to the voltage dependent sodium channels (VDNa$^+$Cs, blue). The VDNa$^+$Cs initiate an action potential that travels along a myelinated axon (yellow) to transmit the pain signal to the brain. B. Cocaine blocks the VDNa$^+$Cs, stopping the transmission of the pain signal. C. An amine pump on the plasma membrane transports the neurotransmitter from the synapse into the presynaptic axon bulb. The pump on the vesicle recycles it for re-release. D. Cocaine blocks the plasma membrane amine pump, allowing the neurotransmitter to build up in the synapse.

to build up in the synapse, hyperstimulating the postsynaptic receptors.

Peripherally, the main effect of this mechanism of action is to inhibit the reuptake of norepinephrine from sympathetic neurons of the autonomic nervous system, mimicking their effects (sympathomimetic). This produces the classic fight-or-flight response: elevated heart rate, increased strength of contraction of the heart, constriction of arteries and veins, dilated bronchial passages, glucose release from the liver, and pupil dilation. The combination of vasoconstriction and cardiostimulation greatly increases blood pressure, which can reach dangerous levels. Vasoconstriction limits the absorption of cocaine through mucous membranes (i.e., when snorting) by limiting blood flow though the tissue. As a result, much of snorted cocaine (up to 70%) is captured by mucus in the nose and drips down the back of the throat. It is then absorbed in the small intestine and mostly destroyed on the first pass through the liver. Vasoconstriction in the nose is responsible for tissue damage in this area, as the tissue becomes necrotic because of the lack of oxygen (see Figure 9.8).

In the CNS, cocaine blocks reuptake transport of dopamine, norepinephrine, and serotonin. The dopamine receptors mainly affected are those in the limbic system (see Figures 5.4 and 5.5). Depending on the rate of absorption, this can produce an intense euphoria, or "rush." This is the effect that is linked to addiction. Norepinephrine-releasing neurons affected by cocaine in the CNS are from the RAS, which initiates stimulation in the brain and produces hyperactivity, excitement, and anorexia. The serotonin-releasing neurons involved are projections from the raphe nucleus. This system is involved with mood; inhibition of serotonin reuptake by cocaine in these neurons produces self-confidence and a sense of well-being.

Thus, the acute central effects of cocaine are euphoria (joy, bordering on giddiness), excitement, and self-confidence. People who use cocaine feel happy, alert, excited, energetic, and full of self-confidence. Cocaine decreases fatigue and appetite. People become very talkative and fun to be around. As the euphoric effects diminish (after ten to thirty minutes), anxiety (due to the hyperstimulation) and craving for more take over. The euphoric effect is limited in time, both because of downregulation of postsynaptic receptors and depletion of the presynaptic nerve terminals of dopamine. The serotonin effect is limited as well and very slow to recover due to slow recovery of depleted serotonin in the nerve terminals. The norepinephrine effect is the most durable response. Users will often continue to take cocaine for the stimulant effects and to avoid the "crash" (see below), long after the other effects have diminished.

Amphetamines

Amphetamines have a similar effect on norepinephrine, dopamine, and serotonin as cocaine

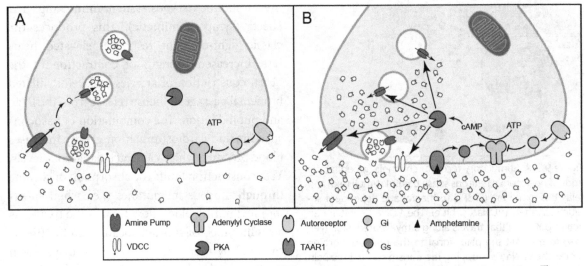

| Amine Pump | Adenylyl Cyclase | Autoreceptor | Gi | Amphetamine |
| VDCC | PKA | TAAR1 | Gs | |

Figure 9.9 A. Under normal conditions, neurotransmitter in the synapse activates the presynaptic autoreceptors. These receptors inhibit the production of cAMP by adenylyl cyclase (by activating G_i), which decreases the amount of neurotransmitter released per action potential. B. Amphetamine stimulates the production of cAMP by binding to the trace amino acid receptor (TAAR1), which activates G_s. cAMP activates protein kinase A (PKA). This phosphorylates the voltage dependent calcium channel (VDCC), increasing the amount of Ca^{2+} entering, increasing synaptic vesicle fusion. In a similar way, proteins kinase C (not shown) is activated and reverses the amine pumps, dumping the neurotransmitter into the synapse.

does, and produce most of the same effects (see Table 9.1), but the mechanism of action is more complicated. Amphetamines both block the reuptake amine pump and reverse it (see Figure 9.8). Amphetamines bind to a receptor on the presynaptic axon bulbs of neurons called the trace amine-associated receptor 1 (TAAR1). TAAR1 is a G-protein coupled receptor that activates G_s to stimulate adenylyl cyclase, increasing cAMP in the axon bulb. This works in opposition to the autoreceptors in these axon bulbs, which decrease neurotransmitter release by inhibiting cAMP production through G_i (see Figure 3.9). Thus, autoreceptors, which respond to neurotransmitter in the synaptic cleft, and TAAR1 modulate the amount of cAMP in the axon bulb.

Elevation of cAMP activates protein kinase A (PKA), which phosphorylates voltage-dependent calcium channels (VDCCs), increasing the influx of calcium during action potentials; this increases vesicle fusion and neurotransmitter release. PKA also phosphorylates the amine pump, causing its internalization, inhibiting its function. In addition, by activating another kinase in the axon bulb (protein kinase C; see Figure 11.4), the amine pump is phosphorylated on a different site, reversing its function. This is true of the amine pump on neurotransmitter storage vesicles as well. This causes the neurotransmitters to be pumped out of the vesicles into the cytoplasm and then out of the cytoplasm into the synapse. The result is a massive release of dopamine, norepinephrine, and serotonin.

The CNS pathways involved and effects produced by amphetamines are the same as those discussed above with cocaine. Dopamine is released in the limbic system, producing a rush of euphoria and addiction; norepinephrine is released in the RAS, producing alertness, excitement, decreased fatigue, and anorexia; serotonin is released by projections from the raphe nucleus, producing confidence and a sense of emotional well-being. The overall effect is a feeling of being powerful, even invincible. Amphetamines are still used in the military in low doses to promote alertness and decrease fatigue and appetite on long flights/missions. However, at high doses they cause extreme euphoria, excitement, and exhilaration and are very addictive.

The main difference between cocaine and amphetamines, as stated before, is the duration of action. An amphetamine high can last twelve hours or more. As with cocaine, the effects produced by dopamine and serotonin diminish, but the norepinephrine effects continue. Withdrawal symptoms following amphetamine use are physically and emotionally painful, so users often re-hit to avoid the crash, remaining awake for days at a time and intensifying the inevitable comedown.

Effects on Cognition

One of the acute effects of amphetamines and cocaine is an increase in attention during tasks. This is one reason why amphetamines are used in the military, especially on long missions. Amphetamines, especially methylphenidate, are used for attention deficit hyperactivity disorder (ADHD). If you recall from Chapter 6, ADHD is a deficit in the ability to deactivate the default-mode network (DMN). There is a lack of anti-correlation between the task-positive network (TPN) and DMN, and, as a result, self-referential thinking intrudes on task performance by the TPN. Amphetamines help restore the balance between the TPN and DMN. Recent fMRI studies show that this is due to effects of dopamine, which is increased by amphetamines and cocaine. Increased dopamine levels decrease connectivity between the anterior cingulate cortex (salience network, SN) and the medial prefrontal cortex (MPC) of the DMN; this increases deactivation of the DMN and shifts cognition to the TPN. Thus, by decreasing functional connectivity between the SN and DMN, amphetamines favor TPN activity, which focuses attention outward.

Adverse Effects
Acute Overdose

Deaths that occur from acute overdose of cocaine or amphetamines are mostly due to the sympathomimetic effects. The vasoconstriction causes ischemia (low blood flow) and hypoxia (lack of oxygen) in tissues (see Figure 9.10). Cell death (tissue necrosis) occurs extensively in the nasal passages due to snorted cocaine, because this is the site of highest cocaine concentration. Cocaine and amphetamines can also cause cerebral ischemia, a condition similar to stroke. This produces brain damage, which decreases memory and can precipitate early onset dementia. In overdose, insufficient cardiac blood flow occurs and causes cardiac cell death. This is produced by the cardiostimulation. Cardiostimulation makes the heart beat stronger and faster, therefore requiring more oxygen. A mismatch between cardiac work and oxygen supply produces cell death and progressive cardiac muscle damage, leading to congestive heart failure. Peripheral necrosis (intestinal, liver, kidney, etc.) is also known to occur due to overdose of cocaine. This is complicated by the fact that the cocaine on the street is sometimes cut with levamisole, a deworming drug that magnifies its vasoconstrictive effects. The sodium channel–blocking properties of cocaine, along with rapid heart rate, can cause arrhythmia and sudden death. The elevated heart rate and strength of heart contraction, together with

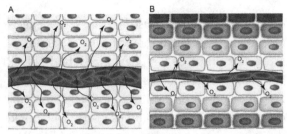

Figure 9.10 A. Each cell in a tissue is within 3 cell widths of a capillary. Under normal situations, oxygen can diffuse this far and satisfy the needs of the cells. B. During cocaine-induced vasoconstriction, there is less blood flow to a tissue (ischemia); this results in less oxygen delivery (hypoxia). Cells receiving insufficient oxygen supply die, leaving necrotic cells (in brown).

peripheral vasoconstriction, can cause extreme high blood pressure, known as hypertensive crisis. Weakened vessels can burst, which is especially dangerous in the case of cerebral hemorrhage (stroke). If high enough, the hypertension can cause aortic rupture and sudden death. Finally, the CNS stimulation through the RAS can precipitate seizures through overstimulation, which can also cause death.

Withdrawal

The short duration of action of cocaine and the craving it induces leads to "coke runs," where the user continually re-doses as the effects diminish. Users snorting cocaine may re-hit every thirty minutes, and crack users every ten minutes, for runs lasting hours to days. Often this is done to avoid the "crash," or withdrawal that quickly follows the decrease in cocaine concentration in the brain.

Withdrawal symptoms are best described as the opposite of the high: extreme tiredness, fatigue, hunger, and depression. Withdrawal can also include anxiety, agitation, and restlessness. The ability to feel pleasure is diminished because of dopamine depletion; ordinary stimuli are no longer enjoyable. Withdrawal from extreme runs of cocaine use can cause body chills and aches, tremors, and shakiness. It also includes strong cravings for more cocaine, often leading to more use and dependence.

Amphetamine users also re-hit to continue the high and avoid withdrawal, although the long half-life means that the interval between doses is greater. The symptoms of the eventual withdrawal are the same as for cocaine but more intense. The often days-long periods of amphetamine abuse seriously deplete dopamine, serotonin, and norepinephrine stores. The depression, fatigue, and anhedonia last longer and are more severe than for amphetamine withdrawal, as is the drug craving.

Tolerance and Dependence

A paradoxical observation for both cocaine and amphetamine is that brief exposure to these drugs cause sensitization rather than desensitization. A single exposure causes a greater response to the drug that can persist for days. However, repeated exposure causes rapid desensitization, especially to the euphoric effects. The reason, as stated above, is because of the depletion of dopamine and serotonin from the nerve terminals as well as downregulation of their receptors. Norepinephrine receptors are also downregulated, but the neurotransmitter itself is more quickly replenished. This leads to a cycle of re-administration to try to recapture the euphoria and avoid withdrawal. The result is a purely stimulatory high, with the concomitant anxiety, paranoia, and anorexia. At its extreme, cocaine or amphetamine addiction produces intense drug craving and compulsive drug taking, as described in Chapter 5. The user is willing to do whatever is necessary to continue using, with no regard for future consequences.

One common feature of the two drugs that encourages dependence is the availability of a nonpolar, freebase form. Crack cocaine and crystal meth are both more addictive than their powdered HCl forms. This is for pharmacokinetic reasons. The fact that these drug forms can be smoked greatly increases their addictive potential. Inhalation is the fastest way to get a drug into the systemic circulation and brain, faster even than IV injection. The rapid increase in brain concentration creates a profound rush of euphoria. The intensity of the rush, which is produced through the limbic system, is directly related to the addictive potential of the drug. As discussed in Chapter 5, this supranormal euphoric stimulus is seen by the PFC as an extremely important event; because of this salience, the PFC reinforces drug-taking behavior through cravings.

Chronic stimulant abuse produces disastrous results in the brain. It precipitates most major psychological disorders, including major depression, anxiety disorder, bipolar disorder, antisocial personality, posttraumatic stress disorder, attention deficit hyperactivity disorder, and psychosis. Symptoms include anxiety, sleeplessness, impulsiveness, repetitive compulsive behaviors, and the inability to sustain interpersonal relationships. Chronic stimulant abuse induces paranoid ideation and persecutory fears; this can lead to a hallucinatory state called toxic paranoid psychosis and aggressive or homicidal behavior. In addition, cocaine abuse usually includes comorbid alcoholism, because alcohol potentiates the effect of cocaine, which makes co-use common.

Methamphetamine is especially known for rapid, premature aging of addicted individuals (see Figure 9.10). Chronic meth users are malnourished due to the anorexia, which gives them a gaunt look. Chronic overstimulation makes their skin itch, a condition called "meth bugs."

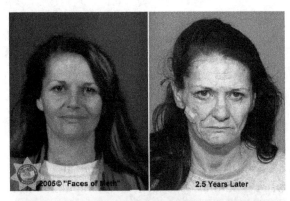

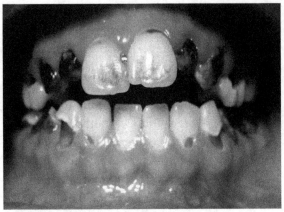

Figure 9.12 Poor personal hygiene, excessive soft drink usage, and the inhibition of saliva production by methamphetamine results in dramatic tooth decay, called "meth mouth."

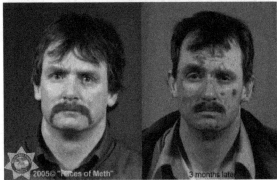

Figure 9.11 Chronic meth users are malnourished, scratch wounds in their skin, and exhibit poor personal hygiene. This causes rapid, premature aging.

This makes them scratch themselves to the point of causing skin lesions; methamphetamine users often have scabs covering their faces and limbs. They practice poor personal hygiene and often drink surgery drinks for energy. This combination, in conjunction with the inhibition of saliva production by methamphetamine, results in dramatic tooth decay, called "meth mouth" (see Figures 9.11 and 9.12). The gaunt look and tooth loss can make a thirty-year-old look like a senior citizen.

Effects on the fetus are also seen in pregnant mothers. Amphetamines and cocaine are fetotoxic, mainly due to vasoconstriction that limits blood flow to the fetus. Placental vessels are constricted, depriving the fetus of oxygen and nutrients. The result is premature or precipitous labor, low birth weight, small head size, and growth retardation.

Disruption of the normal functioning of dopamine, norepinephrine, and serotonin during development may also cause long-term disability. However, the long-term effects of fetal exposure in children born to addicted mothers are difficult to separate from the postnatal effects of the childhood environment. Developmental effects seen in children may also be due to the socioeconomic conditions in a household where drugs are abused: child neglect, lack of maternal attention, poor nutrition and hygiene, and violence in the home.

Summary

There are two major classes of CNS stimulants that are both derived from natural sources. The coca plant is still the primary source of cocaine. Amphetamines were originally derived from the plant product ephedrine (from ma huang) but are now mostly synthetic. Both are amines and can be found in a freebase form, which is heat stable, or an HCl salt form, which is not. The freebase forms are usually smoked, while the

HCl forms are usually snorted or injected. Both of these drugs increase the amount of dopamine, norepinephrine, and serotonin in synapses of the brain. These are neurotransmitters used by the limbic system, reticular activating system, and cells of the raphe nucleus, respectively. The effects produced are euphoria, excitement/stimulation, and a sense of well-being/self-confidence. They main difference in effect is that cocaine is rapidly metabolized and has a very short half-life, approximately fifty minutes. Amphetamines are poorly metabolized and have a half-life of approximately ten hours. The drugs also differ in the way they increase these neurotransmitters; cocaine blocks the mono-amine reuptake pump, while amphetamines activate a trace amino acid receptor (TAAR1) that increases cAMP in the axon bulb and causes both the plasma membrane and vesicular monoamine pumps to reverse. Because both drugs greatly increase dopamine in the limbic system, both are highly addictive. The freebase forms are more addictive because of their rapid absorption through the lungs and distribution to the brain. This produces an intense rush. Acute overdoses occur, mainly due to a sympathomimetic effect produced by the increase of norepinephrine or seizure brought on by over-stimulation of the brain. Chronic abuse results in physical and mental deterioration.

Further Reading

Pharmacokinetics: Jufer R. A., A. Wstadik, S. L. Walsh, B. S. Levine, and E. J. Cone. "Elimination of Cocaine and Metabolites in Plasma, Saliva, and Urine Following Repeated Oral Administration to Human Volunteers." *Journal of Analytical Toxicology* 24 (2000): 467–77.

Cocaine effects: O'Malleya, S., M. Adamseb, R. K. Heatonc, and F. H. Gawina. "Neuropsychological Impairment in Chronic Cocaine Abusers." *The American Journal of Drug and Alcohol Abuse* 18 (1992): 131–44.

Mechanism of amphetamines: Sulzer, D., M. S. Sonders, N. W. Poulsen, and A. Galli. "Mechanisms of Neurotransmitter Release by Amphetamines: A Review." *Progress in Neurobiology* 75 (2005): 406–33.

TAAR1: Grandy, D. K. "Trace Amine-Associated Receptor 1-Family Archetype or Iconoclast?" *Pharmacology and Therapeutics* 116 (2007): 355–90.

Chronic amphetamine abuse: Ornstein, T. J., J. L. Iddon, A. M. Baldacchino, B. J. Sahakian, M. London, B. J. Everitt, and T. W. Robbins. "Profiles of Cognitive Dysfunction in Chronic Amphetamine and Heroin Abusers." *Neuropsychopharmacology* 23 (2000): 113–26.

Stress-related relapse: Mantsch, J. R., O. Vranjkovic, R. C. Twining, P. J. Gasser, J. R. McReynolds, and J. M. Blacktop. "Neurobiological Mechanisms That Contribute to Stress-Related Cocaine Use." *Neuropharmacology* 76 (2014): 383–94.

Cocaine addiction treatment: Fischer, B., P. Blanken, D. Da Silveira, A. Gallassi, E. M. Goldner, J. Rehm, M. Tyndall, and E. Wood. "Effectiveness of Secondary Prevention and Treatment Interventions for Crack-Cocaine Abuse: A Comprehensive Narrative Overview of English-Language Studies." *The International Journal on Drug Policy* 26 (2015): 352–63.

Test Your Understanding
Multiple-Choice

1. This drug is a natural product:
    a. methamphetamine
    b. cocaine
    c. dextroamphetamine
    d. methylphenidate
2. This drug is nonpolar and easily absorbed through mucous membranes:
    a. powder cocaine
    b. powder amphetamine
    c. crystal methamphetamine
    d. all of the above
3. Which of the following has the shortest duration of action?
    a. cocaine HCL
    b. freebase cocaine
    c. methamphetamine HCL
    d. freebase methamphetamine
4. Which of the following is a mechanism of action of cocaine?
    a. local anesthetic
    b. sympathomimetic
    c. psychostimulant
    d. all of the above
5. The neurotransmitter _____ is released by the _____ and produces stimulation.
    a. dopamine, VTA
    b. norepinephrine, RAS
    c. serotonin, raphe nucleus
    d. all of the above
6. What is the source of the addiction of amphetamines and cocaine?
    a. release of dopamine in the NA
    b. release of norepinephrine by the RAS
    c. release of serotonin by the raphe nucleus
    d. all of the above

7. Death from acute effects of amphetamines is usually due to
    a. sympathomimetic effects
    b. inhibition of the medulla and respiratory depression
    c. blocking Na^+ channels in the heart, causing arrhythmia
    d. downregulation of dopamine receptors in the NA
8. Peripheral necrosis
    a. is caused by extreme vasoconstriction
    b. results in "cocaine nose"
    c. is the result of acute ischemia in the affected tissues
    d. all of the above

Essay Questions

1. Compare and contrast cocaine HCl and freebase cocaine. How are they the same? How are they different?
2. Two reasons why cocaine and amphetamines are addictive are because they cause intense cravings and cause compulsive drug use, which are especially intense during withdrawal. Why do these drugs cause cravings and compulsion? What parts of the brain are involved?
3. What is the TAAR1 receptor? What does it do?
4. One of the useful clinical applications of amphetamines, especially methylphenidate, is for ADHD. Why are these drugs effective for this? What mechanism produces this effect?
5. Chronic cocaine users report that they no longer feel the euphoria that was their original draw to the drug. Why is this, based on the mechanism of action of cocaine?

Credits

- Fig. 9.0: Copyright © by Depositphotos / Violin.
- Fig. 9.1a: Copyright © by Depositphotos / jkraft5.
- Fig. 9.1b: Copyright © by Depositphotos / hecke06.
- Fig. 9.4a: Copyright © by Depositphotos / Nomadsoul1.
- Fig. 9.4b: Drug Enforcement Agency / Copyright in the Public Domain.
- Fig. 9.6a: Copyright © by Depositphotos / lekcej.
- Fig. 9.6b: Copyright © 2008 by Radspunk / Wikimedia Commons, (CC BY-SA 4.0) at https://commons.wikimedia.org/wiki/File:Crystal_Meth.jpg.
- Fig. 9.11: Copyright © 2005 by Multnomah County Sheriff's Office. Reprinted with permission.
- Fig. 9.12: Copyright © 2005 by Dozenist / Wikimedia Commons, (CC BY-SA 3.0) at https://commons.wikimedia.org/wiki/File:Suspectedmethmouth09-19-05.jpg.

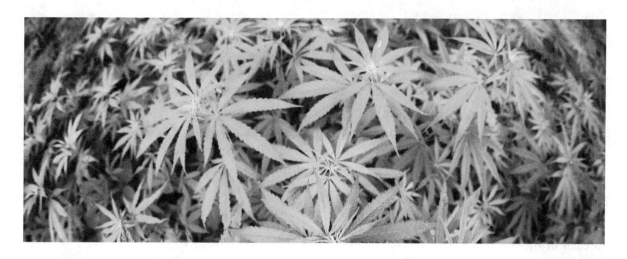

Chapter 10: Cannabis

History

Humans have had a long history with cannabis. Native to central Asia, the plant has been cultivated for more than eight thousand years for its fiber and medicinal qualities. From Asia, its use spread to the Middle East and was widely used throughout the region. Recreational use of cannabis spread through the Roman Empire, but fell off during the Middle Ages.

Cannabis's use as a recreational drug was brought to the West by soldiers of Napoleon's army in the nineteenth century, and it became widespread in France and Europe. Hemp fiber had been widely used in the Western world before this to make rope, fabric, and paper (George Washington famously grew the plant for these purposes), but these strains were very low in psychoactive chemicals.

Recreational use of cannabis was brought to the United States in the early twentieth century by migrants from Mexico, who called it marijuana.

As its use spread through the country, a backlash with strong racist undertones began against it. In the 1930s, the first "drug czar" in the U.S. government, Harry Anslinger, made prohibition of the drug a priority. He began a propaganda campaign based on the erroneous belief that cannabis released subconscious violent tendencies in its users. His effort resulted in the Marihuana Tax Act of 1937. This act made it illegal to buy or sell cannabis without a federal tax stamp (see Figure 10.1); these stamps were sold only to growers of hemp for fiber.

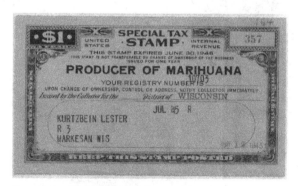

Figure 10.1 The Marihuana Tax Act of 1937 made it illegal to buy or sell cannabis without a federal tax stamp, which were only sold to growers of hemp for fiber.

Cannabis is usually classified into three species, *Cannabis sativa*, *Cannabis indica*, and

Cannabis ruderalis (see Figure 10.2), although it is debated as to whether these are different species or subspecies. Sativa and indica are both cultivated for recreational use. Sativa is the taller of the two, growing to more than six feet in height. Indica is a shorter, thicker plant with broader leaves. Chemically, indica is thought to have a higher tetrahydrocannabinol-to-cannabidiol ratio (these phytochemicals are discussed further below), although individual cultivars can be produced with varying ratios of each of these two active agents. Ruderalis is the least common of the three. This species is small and has very low cannabinoid content. It is adapted to grow and flower quickly in the northern regions of Asia.

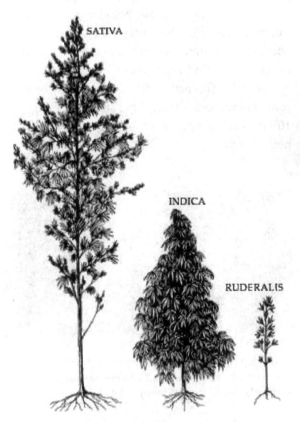

Figure 10.2 The three species of cannabis are C. sativa, C. indica, and C. ruderalis.

Cannabis is dioecious, meaning that male and female sex organs are on separate plants. During cultivation, male plants are weeded out and females are allowed to grow. In this way, the female plants produce flowers that are not allowed to fertilize. This results in buds without seeds, called sinsemilla, that are very high in psychoactive phytochemicals.

Pharmacokinetics

Cannabis is a drug that is commonly used as a whole plant (or more commonly the bud portion of the plant), rather than as a single active ingredient isolated from a plant, as in morphine or cocaine. This is partially because of the ease of use as is, but may also be because there are many active phytochemicals in the plant, and no one phytochemical produces the complete experience. The most commonly recognized active ingredients in cannabis are Δ9-tetrahydrocannabinol (THC) and cannabidiol (CBD). The concentrations of THC and CBD in cannabis are genetically controlled; strains have been developed to produce different concentrations of each and ratios of THC to CBD. In addition, the cannabis bud produces more than sixty other cannabinoids at different concentrations and a range of terpenoids that may also have pharmacological effects. Each strain has its own pharmacological profile, and some of the subjective differences between strains of cannabis may be due to the varied phytochemical constituents of the strains.

Cannabis products are usually bought in one of three different forms. The most common form is the dried bud (see Figure 10.3A). Buds have a frosted appearance due to the many trichomes extending from the surface. A trichome is a glandular, hairlike outgrowth from the leaf, petal, or stem of the plant. THC and other cannabinoids are concentrated in these trichomes (see Figure 10.3B). The concentration of THC in the buds of cannabis plants has increased dramatically since the 1970s. Then the average concentration of THC was between 1 and 3%. Typically consumed buds today average 8.5%, with more potent strains reaching as high as 20%. This increase in concentration increases the dose consumed and the rate of absorption, which has effects on the pharmacology and addictiveness of the drug, as discussed below.

An increase in the THC concentration can easily be achieved by physically removing the trichomes from the bud through rubbing or other

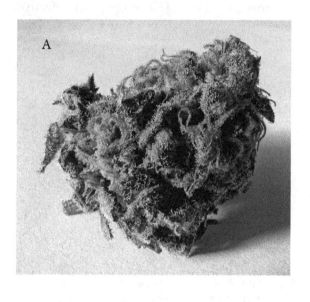

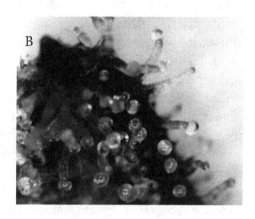

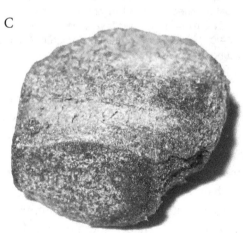

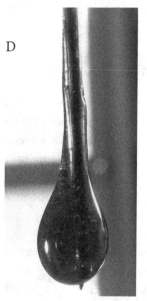

Figure 10.3 A. The dried bud of the female flower is the most popular form of cannabis for recreational use. B. The frosted appearance of the bud is due to the presence of many trichomes extending from the bud. Trichomes have the highest concentration of THC in the plant. C. Hashish is made by physically removing the trichomes and pressing them into a resinous lump. D. Hash oil is made by extracting the cannabinoids from hashish with a nonpolar solvent then evaporating the solvent.

mechanical methods. This concentrated resin material is called hashish, or simply hash (see Figure 10.3C). Depending on the quality, hash can be anywhere from 25 to 65% THC.

Further purification of the active ingredients can be achieved by several different extraction methods. Methods such as dry sieving and ice water extraction physically remove the trichomes to separate them from the rest of the plant material. Chemical separation can be achieved by solvent extraction; this can be done with high-pressure liquid carbon dioxide (CO_2), high-pressure butane, ethyl alcohol, or any organic solvent. After extraction, the solvent is evaporated and an oily resin is left. This method takes advantage of the nonpolar nature of the cannabinoids to separate them from polar chemicals and insoluble plant residue. These methods produce a product of 50 to 90% THC that typically resembles a thick amber liquid or semisolid (see Figure 10.3D), often called hash oil. This is either smoked or vaporized and inhaled.

Absorption and Distribution

Cannabis products are typically consumed by inhalation or oral ingestion, with dramatically different pharmacokinetics for each route (see Figure 10.4). Inhalation is usually done by burning the plant material; the heat from the fire volatilizes the chemicals for inhalation. However, the burning of plant material produces carcinogens (polyaromatic hydrocarbons) and particulates. Safer volatilization techniques (vaping) use an external heat source to volatilize the chemicals without causing ignition of the plant material. The amount of cannabinoids absorbed via inhalation is highly variable (between 2 and 50%) due to personal differences in inhalation (holding in the smoke increases absorption),

but typically averages at about 30%. Cooling the smoke with a water pipe or "bong" concentrates the smoke, increasing the dose per inhalation; it is unclear whether this also removes toxins from the smoke, as studies have produced variable results. Psychoactive effects can be felt quickly after the first inhalation; THC concentration in the plasma peaks in approximately ten minutes. The concentration of THC drops below effective levels in approximately two hours.

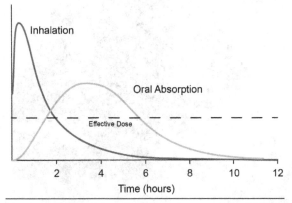

Figure 10.4 After inhalation of smoke containing THC, its concentration peaks in approximately 10 minutes and drops below effective levels in approximately 2 hours. Peak THC from oral absorption is variable with first effects from 30-90 minutes, peaking at approximately 2-3 hours, and lasting from 4-12 hours after onset.

Oral absorption of cannabinoids is much less effective due to poor absorption, stomach degradation, and first-pass metabolism. Bioavailability via oral administration is approximately 4 to 12%. For this reason, a higher dose is usually consumed orally than via inhalation. The increase in THC plasma concentration after oral consumption is delayed, highly variable, and prolonged compared to inhalation. Time to first effect ranges from thirty to ninety minutes, reaching a peak at approximately two to three hours, and can last from four to twelve hours after onset.

Cannabinoids are distributed by the blood via a two-compartment model (see Figure 1.10) and accumulate in fatty tissues. Fatty tissues are a long-term reservoir, and repeated or chronic use of cannabis increases the concentration of lipophilic cannabinoids in the fat over time. Slow diffusion of these cannabinoids out of the fatty tissues decreases potential withdrawal symptoms and increases the length of time between the last use and detection of the metabolites in the urine (see Figure 10.4).

Metabolism and Elimination

The first chemical change that occurs to THC activates it. In the plant, most of the THC is in the carboxyl form tetrahydrocannabinolic acid (THCA; see Figure 10.5A). This is converted to THC (see Figure 10.5B) by heating, either when it is smoked/vaporized or when cooked into edibles. This conversion is necessary to activate THC.

Once consumed, THC is actively metabolized in the liver. After first-pass metabolism of orally consumed THC, only 10% reaches the bloodstream; 10% of it is metabolized to 11-hydroxy-Δ9-tetrahydrocannabinol (11-OH-THC; see Figure 10.5C), which is an active cannabinoid that is more potent than THC. (The conversion to 11-OH-THC happens much more slowly for inhalation and doesn't contribute significantly to the effects of the drug.) The remaining 80% of THC orally consumed is metabolized into 11-nor-9-carboxy-delta-9-tetrahydrocannabinol (carboxy-THC, or THC-COOH; see Figure 10.5D), which is polar and doesn't cross the blood-brain barrier.

Circulating THC and 11-OH-THC are metabolized to THC-COOH in the liver; this effectively inactivates the compound's psychoactive properties and allows the kidneys to excrete it.

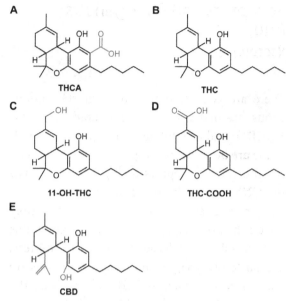

Figure 10.5 A. Tetrahydrocannabinolic acid (THCA) is rapidly converted to THC by heating, which removes the acetate group (in red). B. λ9-tetrahydrocannabinol (THC) is the main psychoactive ingredient in cannabis. C. The liver converts THC to—ΔHydroxy-Δ9-tetrahydrocannabinol (11-OH-THC) by adding a OH group (in blue). D. The liver inactivates the psychoactive effects of THC by adding the carboxy group (in blue), which make the polar compound 11-nor-9-carboxy-delta-9-tetrahydrocannabinol (THC-COOH). E. Cannabidiol (CBD) differs from THC by the functional groups in green.

THC-COOH is the main metabolite used for detection in the urine. The lipophilic compounds THC and 11-OH-THC are stored in fatty tissues and converted into carboxy-THC as they leach out of these tissues and are distributed to the liver. Detection methods for carboxy-THC are very sensitive, and the level of detection of carboxy-THC in urine is extremely low (3 ng/ml, or 3 parts per million). The combination of the slow release of THC and 11-OH-THC from fatty reservoirs and the powerful detection of carboxy-THC combine to allow detection of cannabinoid metabolites for one to two weeks after the last exposure. This can be extended to more than four weeks for users with large fatty deposits who use cannabis chronically.

Receptors and Endogenous Agonists
Receptors

There are two main receptors for the endogenous cannabinoids, cannabinoid receptor 1 (CB1) and cannabinoid receptor 2 (CB2). These are both metabotropic G-protein coupled receptors. CB1 receptors are highly expressed in the CNS, especially in the hippocampus, basal ganglia, cerebellum, and prefrontal cortex. They are on the presynaptic membrane of axon bulbs and inhibit the release of neurotransmitters, similar to presynaptic autoreceptors (see Figure 10.6). Agonists such as THC that activate the CB1 receptors produce the psychotropic effects that are sought by recreational users. For this reason, these will be the main receptors discussed below.

The CB2 receptors are more peripherally located. They are found mainly on cells involved with the immune system, especially leukocytes and cells associated with the lymph glands. They are also found in microglia that perform an immune function in the CNS. These are often the receptors that are targeted by people using medicinal cannabis products (discussed in Box 10.1).

Endogenous Agonists

The effect of THC on the human brain led researchers to search for the receptors for these drugs. In turn, the presence of CB1 and CB2 receptors led to the search for endogenous ligands, which were eventually found. This is called *reverse pharmacology*, going from drug to receptors to endogenous agonist. Historically, the receptors and endogenous agonists were discovered first, followed by the development of drugs that affect them.

The first endogenous agonist found was called anandamide (AEA; see Figure 10.6A), taken from the Sanskrit word for joy or bliss (*ananda*). AEA is a very lipophilic compound made enzymatically through several steps from the twenty-carbon fatty acid arachidonic acid. Arachidonic acid is a common component of membrane phospholipids that is released from diacylglycerol (DAG) by the activity of diacylglycerol lipase (DAGL). AEA is a partial agonist of CB1 receptors, activating them but not fully. It is even less active at CB2 receptors, being a partial agonist to antagonist. The second endocannabinoid discovered was 2-arachidonoyl glycerol (2-AG). 2-AG has a similar structure to AEA, with a glycerol group replacing the ethanolamine group (see Figure 10.6B). 2-AG is a full agonist at both CB1 and CB2 receptors. In addition, the brain

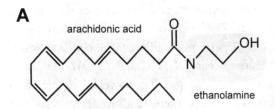

Anandamide

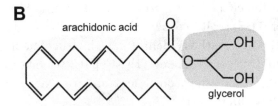

2- Arachidonoyl glycerol

Figure 10.6 A. Anandamide was the first endocannabinoid discovered. It is a partial agonist at CB1 and CB2 receptors. B. 2-Arachidonoyl glycerol is a full agonist at CB1 and CB2 receptors. These molecules are made from arachidonic acid (in yellow) combined with either ethanolamine (in blue) for AEA or glycerol (in pink) for 2-AG.

There has been much recent attention to the medicinal use of cannabis, although it has been used this way for centuries. Many states have legalized its prescription by licensed physicians for different medical conditions, and much research has recently been conducted showing benefits in a number of disorders.

The medicinal effects are partly through activation of CB2 receptors by CBD. One therapeutic target with CB2 receptors is the leukocyte. Leukocytes release locally active hormones that produce inflammation, swelling, and pain. Like CB1 receptors (see Figure 10.7), CB2 receptors are coupled to G_i. In leukocytes, activation of CB2 receptors inhibits cAMP production and produces K^+ channel activation, as in neurons. This inhibits the immune response of leukocytes, relieving the inflammation and pain. This inhibition is important to the anti-inflammatory and analgesic effects of CB2 receptor agonists.

CB2 receptors in the CNS are found on microglia in the PFC. These support cells perform an immune function in the brain. There is evidence that agonists of CB2 receptors can produce neuroprotection against degenerative diseases such as Huntington's and Parkinson's diseases, presumably though their inhibitory action on microglia.

There are also beneficial therapeutic effects of activation CB1 receptors with the agonist THC. THC has anti-seizure properties and is effective in treating neurogenic pain (i.e., pain cause by hyperactive neurons). For this reason, it and can be effective in multiple sclerosis and childhood epilepsy. In addition, THC is anxiolytic and has a central analgesic effect. THC has central effects on appetite; Marinol (synthetic THC) is used to inhibit nausea and increase appetite in AIDS and cancer treatment. CBD is often added to medicinal THC preparations in a one-to-one mixture. CBD is a CB1 receptor antagonist, and it moderates the psychotropic effects of THC, which can limit its daily use. Finally, CBD has been suggested to be useful as an antipsychotic. As a CB1 receptor antagonist, CBD can block glutamate excitotoxicity and excessive synaptic pruning (however, this use is speculative).

Thus, there are many possible uses of cannabinoid drugs. Recently, there has been a more liberal attitude toward research with cannabinoids, which may help develop treatments for the disorders mentioned above and others.

releases much more 2-AG than AEA, which suggests that it is the major endogenous agonist of the CB1 receptor. Three other endogenous chemicals have been found that are also active at CB receptors, but are produced at much lower concentrations.

Endocannabinoids are different from most neurotransmitters in that they are not premade, stored in vesicles, and release by exocytosis; they are made by enzymes in the postsynaptic membrane as they are needed (see Figure 10.7). Because they are lipophilic, they diffuse out of the releasing cell and across the synapse to the receiving cell. A second major difference is that they are one of the few neurotransmitters that are released by the postsynaptic cell and received by the presynaptic cell. To terminate transmission, the endocannabinoid is transported back into the postsynaptic membrane. This is called *retrograde transmission*, in that it is the opposite of what is seen in almost every other neurotransmitter. Inside the postsynaptic membrane, endocannabinoids are hydrolyzed by specific enzymes. AEA is hydrolyzed by fatty acid amide hydrolase (FAAH), and 2-AG is hydrolyzed by monoacylglycerol lipase (MAGL) as well FAAH.

Mechanism of Action

Activated CB1 receptors in the presynaptic membrane are linked through G_i to inhibition of cAMP production, activation of K^+ channels, and inhibition of voltage-dependent calcium channels (see Figure 10.7). This is similar to the mechanism of action of μ opiate receptors (see Chapter 8). All three of these mechanisms decrease the amount of Ca^{2+} entering during an action potential, leading to a decrease in the amount of neurotransmitter released by the presynaptic axon bulb. CB1 receptors have been shown to decrease the release of the excitatory neurotransmitters glutamate and acetylcholine, as well as the neurotransmitter norepinephrine in the cortex. They are also linked to inhibition of GABA release in the hippocampus.

Endogenous Effects

CB1 receptors are widely expressed in the CNS, and, therefore, there are many functions of endocannabinoids (see Table 10.1). There are high concentrations of these receptors in areas involved in cognition, mood, memory, pain perception, and motor control.

CB1 receptors are expressed densely in many areas of the cerebral cortex, including the medial prefrontal cortex (MPC), anterior cingulate cortex (ACC), posterior cingulate cortex (PCC), insula, and precuneus. These are all regions that are important in the default-mode network

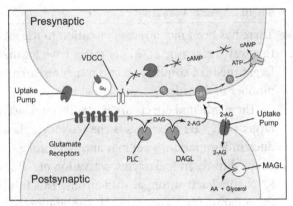

Figure 10.7 Mechanism of Action of Endocannabinoids. Phosphatidylinositol (PI, center) is converted into diacylglycerol by phospholipase C (PLC); this is converted to 2-AG by diacylglycerol lipase (DAGL). 2-AG diffuses retrograde across the synapse and activates the CB1 receptor. CB1 receptors are linked to inhibition of cAMP production through G_i, inhibition of the voltage dependent calcium channel (VDCC) through Gq, and activation of K^+ channels (not shown). These actions inhibit the VDCC, which decreases Ca^{2+} entry and glutamate (Glu release). 2-AG is pumped back into the post synaptic membrane and broken down by monoacylglycerol lipase (MAGL) to halt transmission.

(DMN) and salience network (SN) discussed in Chapter 6. Endocannabinoids may be important in modulating cognition, favoring the activation of DMN and creative thought, but inhibiting salience processing by inhibition of the ACC.

CB1 receptors are important for processing emotions. Emotional processing involves connections between the limbic system (especially the amygdala, where CB1 receptors are dense) and the MPC (part of the DMN). CB1 receptors here modulate neuroplasticity in the amygdala and MPC based on the emotional salience of events. Neuroplasticity is important for long-term memories based on the significance of the event. Endocannabinoids decrease fear processing, making them anxiolytic. They also increase association with positive emotions. In general, activation of CB1 receptors produces a relaxed state and calms aggressive behaviors. There is evidence that

Table 10.1 Comparison of endogenous and recreational effects of CB1 receptor activation

CB1 Receptor Location	Endogenous Effect	Recreational Dose
MPC, PCC, and precuneus	Default-mode processing Mind wandering and creative thought	Altered sense of reality, dream-like state Increase in mind wandering and creative thought Mental confusion (high dose)
ACC and insula	Salience processing Controlled focus Favoring of DMN	Decreased ability to focus Concentration deficits
Amygdala and MPC	Emotional processing Anxiolytic effect (decreases fear response) Decrease in fearful memories Calming of aggressive behavior	Calming of aggressive behavior Anxiolytic effect Anxiety/paranoia at high doses
Hippocampus and PCC	Short- to long-term memory processing Resetting the hippocampus	Decrease in short-term memory
Basal ganglia, cerebellum, MPC	Fine motor coordination Time perception	Disrupted motor coordination Reduced time perception
Hypothalamus and NA	Inhibition of leptin, potentiation of orexin Increased food craving, dulled sense of fullness	Increased appetite
NA and VTA	Slight euphoria	Moderate euphoria Addiction potential
PAG and DRG	Modulation of pain	Decreased pain

cannabinoids may be involved in the extinction of conditioned fear (i.e., losing a fearful feeling that builds up in response to repetitive negative stimuli). This line of evidence suggests that cannabinoids may someday be useful in treating posttraumatic stress disorder (PTSD).

Another functional link with a high concentration of CB1 receptors is the hippocampus-to-PCC pathway. As discussed in Chapter 6, the hippocampus is functionally connected to the PCC, which is part of the DMN. The hippocampus is the part of the limbic system that provides short-term memory, and the PCC provides a connection between the limbic system and the cortex. The PCC measures the emotional salience of events and passes them to the MPC for conscious awareness. It also helps transfer emotionally salient short-term memories in the hippocampus into long-term memories in the

cortex during sleep; the hippocampus is then reset to receive new memories the following day. Endocannabinoids are involved in the process of resetting the hippocampus overnight. CB1 receptors in the hippocampus are found on both the GABAergic and glutaminergic neurons, causing inhibition of release in both cases. GABAergic neurons inhibit and glutaminergic neurons enhance learning and memory. Thus, local control of neurotransmitter release by endocannabinoids is important for proper memory function.

CB1 receptors are highly expressed in the basal ganglia (substantia nigra) and moderately expressed in the cerebellum. These regions modulate fine motor coordination. Smooth movements, such as those performed in athletic or dance moves, require rapid, coordinated contraction and relaxation of many muscles at the same time. They also involve timely corrections based on changes in balance and body position. Timing is an associated role of this process. The cerebellum coordinates with the MPC to ensure that movements happen with the correct timing. You can imagine the importance of split-second timing in the proper execution of a perfect lay-up in basketball; all movements must be perfect to complete the task. The expression of CB1 receptors in the basal ganglia and cerebellum suggests that endocannabinoids play an important role in fine-tuning these movements.

CB1 receptors expressed in the thalamus and nucleus accumbens are important in the regulation of food intake (see Figure 10.8). Food intake is affected by three peptide hormones: leptin, ghrelin, and orexin. Leptin is a hormone released by adipose tissue and the stomach; it activates the sensation of being full and inhibits hunger sensation through actions in the hypothalamus in order to regulate appetite. Ghrelin does the opposite; it is also released by the stomach and inhibits the effects of leptin on the hypothalamus to increase hunger. Orexin is a central control of hunger; it is released within the hypothalamus in response to hypoglycemia. It increases cravings for food and decreases the sense of fullness. It also is important for wakefulness, waking a person up when he or she is hypoglycemic.

Activation of CB1 receptors in the hypothalamus inhibits the effect of leptin, increasing hunger sensation. CB1 receptors also work synergistically with orexin. Orexin-releasing neurons are inhibited by leptin and activated by endocannabinoids and ghrelin. Thus, endocannabinoids are intimately linked with increasing appetite and food intake through receptors in the hypothalamus.

Expression of CB1 receptors in the limbic system includes moderate expression in the nucleus accumbens (NA) and dense expression in the amygdala. In addition, CB1 receptors modulate

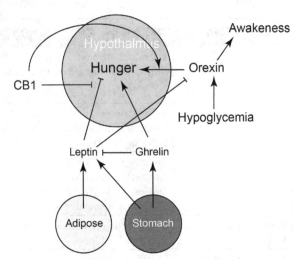

Figure 10.8 Leptin, released by adipose cells and the stomach, inhibits the hunger sensation in the hypothalamus. Orexin, released centrally due to hypoglycemia, increases hunger sensation and produces excitement, arousal. Ghrelin inhibits the effect of leptin and directly stimulates the hypothalamus, increasing hunger sensation. CB1 receptors in the hypothalamus block the effects of leptin and augment the effects of orexin, increasing cravings for food and decreasing the sense of fullness.

both glutaminergic and GABAergic input into the ventral tegmental area (VTA); these neurons project dopamine-releasing neurons into the limbic system. The CB1 receptors in the NA are linked to neurons in the hypothalamus that receive leptin input; leptin increases activation of these receptors, producing reward after eating. CB1 receptors in the NA and VTA, in general, produce mild euphoria by increasing dopamine release. This produces mild reward after eating a meal. This can lead to addiction in the abuse of cannabinoids, as discussed below.

In terms of pain modulation, CB1 receptors are highly expressed in the same areas where μ opioid receptors modulate pain. This includes the central control region of the periaqueductal gray region (PAG) as well as the spinal cord at the dorsal root ganglia (DRG). Endocannabinoids work synergistically with endorphins and enkephalins, enhancing their inhibiting effect on the perception of painful stimuli.

In general, endocannabinoids provide modulation of brain activity, especially in emotional processing (increasing positive emotions), memory (decreasing memory, resetting the hippocampus), movement control (increasing smoothness and timing of movements), appetite regulation (increasing appetite), and default-mode cognition (increasing cognition). You can imagine this as sporadic, low-level tweaking of cognition to make it more precise and efficient.

Recreational Effects

CB1 receptor agonists, such as THC and 11-OH-THC, produce the same effects in neurons as endocannabinoids do. The main difference is the level of receptor activation (high) and duration of the effect (long). Endocannabinoids are released locally (in one area of the brain at a time) at low levels and are quickly degraded. Each individual site is controlled separately, based on the physiological function of that synapse alone. Exogenous agonists, such as THC, are taken in large doses that maximally activate all CB1 receptors. Also, their effects last for hours, continuing until the agonists are transported to the liver and metabolized. The difference between endogenous cannabinoid effects and recreational doses can be likened to the difference between watering certain plants in your garden and experiencing a flooding downpour that drenches the whole yard.

Unlike many other drugs, the effects of cannabis intoxication can be very subjective; the experience is affected by the person's emotional state, the setting where the drug is taken, and previous experiences with the drug. Drugs such as cocaine, amphetamines, and opiates, which produce their main affects in lower, more primitive areas of the brain, are more consistent in effect in different people. Drugs such as THC and hallucinogens affect higher levels of the brain that are involved in cognition, which is much more complicated. For this reason, it is more difficult for one person to convey the cannabis experience to another. However, in general terms, cannabis distorts a person's sense of reality, producing a dream-like state. It enhances visual, auditory, and gustatory (taste) perception, and distorts time perception. It negatively affects concentration (task-positive mode, TPN), and enhances free-floating, fanciful thinking (DMN). Cannabis decreases aggressive behavior, causes a moderate euphoric sensation, and produces an overall sense of well-being.

The most consistently measured effect of THC is cognitive disruption; studies of focused concentration while high show serious cognitive deficits. Overstimulating the CB1 receptors in the MPC and ACC favors DMN processing and inhibits proper salience processing (see Figure 10.9). As a result, there is significantly less anti-correlation between TPN and DMN when a person is trying to focus on a task while high. The DMN is especially important for mind wandering, which is linked to creative thinking. However, the negative correlation with focused concentration makes it difficult to act on this creativity to complete a project, which is done by TPN processing. In addition, overstimulation of CB1 receptors in the hippocampus inhibits short- and long-term memory formation. These cognitive deficits may come with the trade-off of increased creativity, although studies on this are mixed. Some studies show increases in creativity at low doses, and some show no effect. However, all studies show a decrease in creativity at high doses, possibly due to the mental confusion common at high doses (see below).

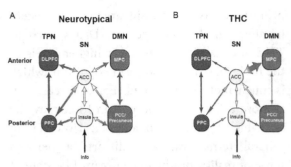

Figure 10.9 A. This is a schematic representation of normal processing of cognition, reproduced from Chapter 6. B. THC causes an increase of activity in the medial prefrontal cortex (MPC) and inhibits salience network (SN) processing by the anterior cingulate cortex (ACC), increasing default mode network (DMN) processing. This causes de-emphasis of the dorsolateral prefrontal cortex (DLPC), which is important for focused attention. At high doses THC can inhibit processing within the DMN, between the MPC and posterior cingulate cortex (PCC)/precuneus, which produces depersonalization.

Perception of time in the human brain involves functional connectivity among the ACC, basal ganglia, cerebellum, and MPC. Time is judged by a cerebellar-MPC pathway. All of these regions are endowed with moderate to dense concentrations of CB1 receptors. Overstimulation of these receptors with THC disrupts their function and inhibits the ability to estimate time. This is well established and is often used by law enforcement as a basis of road sobriety tests.

Low doses of THC are anxiolytic, most likely because of effects on the amygdala and the amygdala/MPC pathway, which are rich in CB1 receptors. Low doses also release dopamine in the NA, causing mild euphoria. Together these effects produce a mellow, happy, relaxed feeling. However, high doses of THC have the opposite effect, producing anxiety and paranoia. This may be due to receptors other than cannabinoid receptors (e.g., vanilloid receptors) that have a lower affinity for THC and become activated at higher doses.

Cannabis is well known for causing an increase in appetite. As of this writing, the only

FDA-approved use of Marinol (THC tablets) is for treating the loss of appetite that accompanies AIDS and chemotherapy. The effect on appetite is due to the CB1 receptors in the thalamus that modulate its response to leptin (discussed above). This simulates a starvation response, activating hunger and blocking satiety (i.e., it causes "the munchies").

THC overstimulation of CB1 receptors in the motor control areas (basal ganglia and cerebellum) disrupts coordinated movement. This effect, combined with the disruption of cerebellum-controlled timing and lack of attention due to inhibition of the SN (i.e., inability to switch to TPN efficiently), makes driving dangerous. It is even more dangerous when combined with alcohol (which is common), because both of these drugs decrease reaction time and inhibit motor coordination.

Negative Effects
Risk of Overdose

Compared to other Schedule I drugs, THC is very safe (see Figure 10.10). Safety is determined by the therapeutic index (TI) of drugs. *TI is the ratio of the effective dose of the drug to the toxic or lethal dose.* For a drug with a narrow therapeutic window, such as heroin, the TI can be as small as a two- to threefold difference between getting high and overdose. The commonly used drug alcohol has a five- to tenfold difference between a pleasurable experience and toxicity. For the relatively safe drug caffeine, this difference is one-hundredfold. For cannabis, the difference is one-thousandfold. It is very difficult to inject this much cannabis into the body. The main danger in high-dose cannabis occurs when people get high and then engage in risky behavior, such as

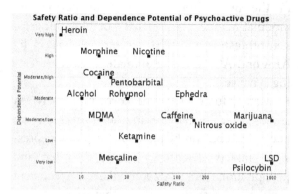

Figure 10.10 Relative Safety and Addictive Potential of Recreational Drugs. This graph shows the relative safety and addictiveness of recreational drugs. Safety is determined by the ratio of effective dose to toxic dose. The safest drugs have the widest margin of safety, on the far right of the graph. Addictiveness is determined by the capture ratio, which is the ratio of the number of people who try a drug vs. the number who become habitual or addicted users. The most addictive drugs are at the top of the scale.

driving a car or performing dangerous athletic stunts. This is because of the combination of cognitive disruption, time distortion, and physical inhibition.

Acute High Dose: Cognitive Confusion

Despite the relative safety of cannabis, at very high doses, it can have very unpleasant effects, especially the induction of anxiety and paranoia. This may be due to effects at lower-affinity, non-cannabinoid receptors, as mentioned above. It also produces cognitive confusion because of effects on the ACC, which is a central hub of the SN, and on the MPC, which is part of the DMN. Cognitive confusion may be part of a phenomenon called "ego depletion." Overstimulation of CB1 receptors (and possibly other receptors) overwhelms the brain's resources, and the person is unable to exert control over thinking. This causes a stupor-like state, where the person is

unable to respond to the environment intelligently. Inhibition of the motor control areas (basal ganglia and cerebellum) contributes to physical inhibition (sedation and inactivity). This is accompanied by a sight depersonalization, or loss of sense of self. The sense of self (which will be discussed more in Chapter 11) is a function of the DMN, coordinating between the precuneus and the MPC. If the DMN is disrupted enough, this processing can be lost, producing depersonalization. Finally, hallucinations may be produced at extreme doses because of overstimulation of the primary and secondary sensory cortex (especially visually) and the inability of the executive functioning to control these regions.

Tolerance and Dependence

Traditionally, cannabis has been considered less likely to produce tolerance or dependence than many other drugs (see Figure 10.10). This is due to a number of factors that differentiate it from classically addictive drugs, such as cocaine or opiates. One difference is the lipid solubility of THC and 11-OH-THC. A low concentration of these persists in the blood and brain for days or weeks after use is terminated. This creates a condition called *reverse tolerance*, where later doses of the drug seem more potent because there is already a significant concentration of THC in the blood during re-administration. Also, the slow removal creates a weaning effect. This decreases the incidence of withdrawal symptoms that are commonly seen in drugs that are rapidly removed from the brain.

However, newer, more potent strains of cannabis may change this relationship. The higher THC concentration causes a higher and faster peak of THC effect in the brain, which includes the production of increased euphoria through stimulation of the NA and VTA. This is the pleasure-circuit mechanism that all addictive drugs share. High-potency cannabis produces a greater rush than lower-potency cannabis does and increases its addiction potential. As a result, an abstinence syndrome (withdrawal) can be seen in chronic, high-dose users who become suddenly abstinent. Withdrawal symptoms include cravings for cannabis, anxiety, sleeplessness, irritability, depression, and appetite suppression. While these symptoms are uncomfortable and often lead to relapse, they are much milder than those seen with harder drugs (e.g., alcohol and opiates).

CB1 Receptors and Adolescent Development

Adolescence is the period between puberty and adulthood. It is a period of physical and psychological maturation, generally occurring in the late teen years. Psychological maturation involves remodeling of the brain, especially the PFC areas involved in decision making, emotional processing, and risk taking (central to the role of the MPC, part of the DMN) and areas involved in foresight and planning (dorsolateral PFC, part of the TPN). This remodeling causes the development of improved impulse control (inhibition of the limbic system) and better evaluation of risks and rewards. Maturation is paradoxically produced by a reduction in gray matter, rather than growth of new neurons (see Figure 10.11). Neurons are removed and cognition is streamlined by a process called *synaptic pruning*. Unused pathways are removed and active pathways are strengthened. The strengthened pathways experience increased myelination, increasing their efficiency. This process begins in early adolescence in sensory and motor regions and then proceeds to the PFC.

Synaptic pruning is modulated by the endocannabinoid system. CB1 receptors are expressed in the brain from the prenatal period on, modulating the excitotoxicity of glutaminergic neurotransmission. CB1 receptor activation by AEA or 2-AG inhibits glutamate release, protecting synapses.

Many studies show a correlation between adolescent cannabis use and later psychological and emotional problems. This includes depression, anxiety disorders, bipolar disorder, and precipitation of schizophrenia. A recurrent problem with these studies is that they are typically cross-sectional studies. Chronic users and abstinent control subjects are matched for age, gender, and duration of use and comparisons are made between the two groups. Few studies, however, are designed to show longitudinal changes (changes in individuals over time). This creates a chicken-and-the-egg problem. Are the differences seen in chronic users because of their exposure to cannabis, or are individuals with these structural differences self-medicating with cannabis? At this point, we do not yet have an answer to this question. But the importance of CB1 receptors in neuroadaptation and synaptic pruning in development at this age suggests that it would be prudent to avoid cannabis until adulthood.

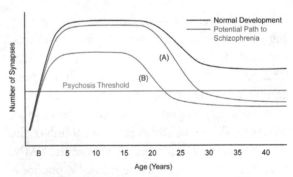

Figure 10.11 This figure hypothesizes two possible routes to psychosis. Normal neurodevelopment involves a decrease in synaptic connectivity in the adolescent years. Schizophrenia is caused by less synaptic connectivity than normal. This may be due to over pruning during adolescence (A) or a lower original baseline of connectivity before adolescence (B).

Changes in Chronic Use

Many studies have been performed in humans to determine structural and functional differences between the brains of abstinent individuals and those who use cannabis long-term. CB1 receptor downregulation is seen in the areas where these receptors are most dense: the amygdala, hippocampus, MPC, insula, ACC, and NA. Structural changes are seen in these areas as well. While the studies are often contradictory (some show increases and others show decreases in the same area), one consistent result is a decrease in gray matter (cell bodies) in the MPC and an increase in white matter (axon tracts). This accompanies an increase in resting-state functional connectivity of the MPC (see Figure 10.12). This includes the MPC-amygdala pathway, which is important in emotional processing, motivation, and decision making. The decreases in gray matter suggests a deficit in memory and executive processing, while the increase in MPC connectivity suggests increased DMN activation. This correlates well with decades of studies showing impairment in decision making, memory, and focus in chronic cannabis users.

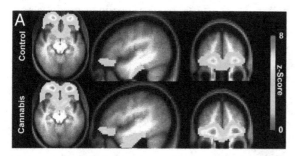

Figure 10.12 This figure shows functional connectivity maps of controls and cannabis users. Note the increases in activity in the medial prefrontal cortex in cannabis users. (Reprinted from Filbey et. al., PNAS 111(47) p. 16915.)

Depression is a common mental illness associated with emotional processing. Some studies suggest that it is linked to increased MPC functional connectivity with the amygdala (see Chapter 6). Because chronic cannabis use is associated with increases in MPC activation, one might assume that it could also be associated with depression. Depression is commonly seen in chronic cannabis use and is often diagnosed as amotivational syndrome. Amotivational syndrome is marked by sustained apathy, poor short-term memory, disinterest in pursing long-term goals, and reluctance to engage in social activities. As discussed above, it is yet unclear whether chronic cannabis use is a cause or a symptom of amotivational syndrome; however, it is commonly associated with cannabis.

Schizophrenia

Schizophrenia is a neurodevelopmental disorder that is characterized by an inability to distinguish between what is real and imaginary. There are many different expressions of this disease, including any or all of the following: visual and auditory hallucinations, persecutory fears (paranoia), delusional thinking, disorganized speech, and lack of motivation. Schizophrenia typically appears during adolescent development and shortly thereafter (between sixteen and thirty years of age) and rarely appears after age forty, suggesting a role of development in its expression. The causes are varied, with both genetic and environmental influences. For example, the enzyme catechol-O-methyl transferase, which breaks down dopamine, is often mutated in schizophrenics and is a potential genetic marker. Also, childhood trauma is associated with schizophrenia, showing the importance of the developmental environment.

One neurological cause of schizophrenia is abnormal synaptic pruning during development (see Figure 10.11). Schizophrenics have decreased gray matter in cortical regions compared to normal controls. Many lines of evidence show that this loss of gray matter is due to excessive synaptic pruning. The importance of endocannabinoids in synaptic pruning suggests that chronic use of cannabis during development may affect the expression of this disease. Indeed, a connection between adolescent cannabis use and first psychotic break has been established. The progression of the disease in susceptible individuals has been shown to be accelerated by chronic use, especially when the onset of use is early and high-potency strains are used. Newer high-potency strains tend to have a lower CBD content; CBD plays a protective role by blocking CB1 receptors and may even help alleviate psychotic symptoms. However, while cannabis use has been shown to precipitate the first psychotic break in susceptible individuals, it has not been shown to cause schizophrenia in individuals not otherwise prone to its expression.

Summary

Cannabis use and cultivation have been part of the human experience since the beginnings of civilization. Cannabis has had medicinal and recreational uses, in addition to supplying an important source of fiber for rope and clothing. Recreational use expanded in the twentieth century, which resulted in a large commercial market for the drug and its prohibition. The two main active ingredients in cannabis are THC and CBD. These are agonists of the CB1 and CB2 receptors, respectively. CB1 receptors are mainly found in the CNS and are linked to the psychotropic and some of the medical effects of cannabis. CB2 receptors are not psychotropic and are mainly peripheral; they are linked to the remainder of the medicinal uses of cannabis. CB1 receptors are found on the presynaptic membranes of axon bulbs. They are metabotropic, activating G-proteins that inhibit cAMP production, block voltage-dependent calcium channels, and open K^+ channels, all of which inhibit the neurotransmitter release. The endogenous agonists for CB1 and CB2 receptors are AEA and 2-AG. These are nontraditional neurotransmitters; they are synthesized in the postsynaptic neuron immediately prior to release, travel to the presynaptic neuron to activate receptors, and are taken up by the postsynaptic neuron to be degraded. These endogenous neurotransmitters are important in DMN activity, salience processing, emotional processing, memory, fine motor coordination, appetite control, and pain modulation. These effects are produced by receptors in the MPC, ACC, PCC, precuneus, amygdala, hippocampus, basal ganglia, cerebellum, thalamus, NA, and PAG. Recreational use overstimulates these receptors and distorts a person's sense of reality, producing a dream-like state. It enhances visual, auditory, and taste perception and distorts the sense of time and time perception. It negatively affects concentration, leading to free-floating, fanciful thinking. Cannabis decreases aggressive behavior, causes a moderate euphoric sensation, and produces an overall sense of well-being. Extreme doses can produce anxiety and paranoia. Chronic use is associated with changes in cortical gray and white matter, although cause and effect are unclear. Adolescent use is associated with mood disorders and should be strongly discouraged.

Further Reading

Pharmacokinetics: Huestis, Marilyn A. "Human Cannabinoid Pharmacokinetics." *Chemistry & Biodiversity* 4 (2007): 1770–804.

Grotenhermen, F. "Pharmacokinetics and Pharmacodynamics of Cannabinoids." *Clinical Pharmacokinetics* 42 (2003): 327–60.

Mechanism of action: Kofalvi, A., R. J. Rodrigues, C. Ledent, K. Mackie, S. Vizi, R. A. Cunha, and B. Sperlagh. "Involvement of Cannabinoid Receptors in the Regulation of Neurotransmitter Release in the Rodent Striatum: A Combined Immunochemical and Pharmacological Analysis." *Journal of Neuroscience* 25 (2005): 2874–84.

Svíženskáa, I., P. Dubovýa, A. and Šulcováb. "Cannabinoid Receptors 1 and 2 (CB1 and CB2), Their Distribution, Ligands and Functional Involvement in Nervous System Structures—A Short Review." *Pharmacology Biochemistry and Behavior* 90 (2008): 501–11.

Endogenous signaling: Wilson, R. I., and R. A. Nicoll. "Endogenous Cannabinoids Mediate Retrograde Signaling at Hippocampal Synapses." Nature 410 (2001): 588–92.

Neuroimaging: Martı́n-Santos, R., A. B. Fagundo, J. A. Crippa1, Z. Atakan, S. Bhattacharyya, P. Allen, P. Fusar-Poli, S. Borgwardt, M. Seal, G. F. Busatto, and P. McGuire. "Neuroimaging in Cannabis Use: A Systematic Review of the Literature." *Psychological Medicine* 40 (2010): 383–98.

Chronic effects: Filbeya, F. M., S. Aslana, V. D. Calhounc, J. S. Spencea, E. Damarajuc, A. Caprihanc, and J. Segallc. "Long-Term Effects of Marijuana Use on the Brain." *Proceedings of the National Academy of Sciences* 111 (2014): 16913–8.

Schizophrenia: Di Forti, M., C. Morgan, P. Dazzan, C. Pariante, V. Mondelli, T. Reis Marques, R. Handley, S. Luzi, M. Russo, and A. Paparelli. "High-Potency Cannabis and the Risk of Psychosis." *British Journal of Psychiatry* 195 (2009): 488–91.

Test Your Understanding
Multiple-Choice

1. The tallest species of the cannabis family is
   a. *Cannabis sativa*
   b. *Cannabis indica*
   c. *Cannabis ruderalis*
   d. *Cannabis sinsemilla*
2. Which cannabis product has the highest concentration of active ingredients?
   a. dried buds
   b. isolated trichomes
   c. hashish
   d. hash oil
3. The main cannabinoid metabolite excreted in the urine is
   a. THCA
   b. THC
   c. 11-OH-THC
   d. THC-COOH
4. Match the cannabinoid with its receptor (select the two correct answers):
   a. THC—CB2
   b. THC—CB1
   c. CBD—CB1
   d. CBD—CB2
5. The main endocannabinoid release in the brain is
   a. AEA
   b. 2-AG
   c. THC
   d. CDB

6. THC in the cortex tends to favor which type of cognition?
   a. DMN
   b. TPM
   c. SN
   d. all of the above

7. The effects of THC on short-term memory are due to
   a. the amygdala-MPC pathway
   b. the PCC-hippocampus pathway
   c. the MPC-basal ganglia/cerebellum pathway
   d. the hypothalamic orexin/ghrelin/leptin pathway

8. The distortion of time produced by THC is due to
   a. the amygdala-MPC pathway
   b. the PCC-hippocampus pathway
   c. the MPC-basal ganglia/cerebellum pathway
   d. the hypothalamic orexin/ghrelin/leptin pathway

Essay Questions

1. Describe three ways in which orally ingesting cannabis products is different from inhalation.

2. Describe the production, release, removal from the synapse, and metabolism of 2-AG.

3. What is the mechanism that CB1 receptors use to produce their effects?

4. Why has it been suggested that cannabis may be useful for PTSD?

5. What differences are seen in brain scans of chronic users of cannabis? How does this relate to the stereotype of chronic users?

Credits

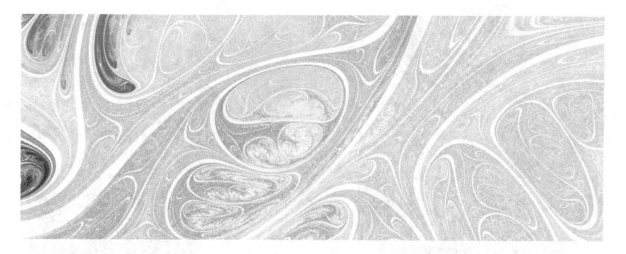

Chapter 11: Hallucinogens

Categories of Hallucinogens

There are four main classes of hallucinogens, based on their mechanism of action and effects. The most familiar are the psychedelics. These include the drugs lysergic acid diethylamide (LSD), psilocybin, and dimethyltryptamine (DMT). A second class is the dissociative anesthetics, which were originally developed for surgery. The main drugs in this class are phencyclidine (PCP) and ketamine. The third class are deliriants, which are anti-muscarinic drugs, such as atropine and scopolamine. The fourth class is called stimulant hallucinogens. The main drugs of this class are 3,4-methylenedioxymethamphetamine (MDMA) and mescaline. Each of these classes of drugs is considered separately in this chapter.

Psychedelics

History

The word *psychedelic* is derived from the Greek for "mind-revealing." They are also called *entheogenic*, which is Greek for "generating the God within." This is reflected in their historic use in religious and medicinal rituals. The shaman or patient would imbibe the psychoactive in an attempt to contact an alternate reality where answers could be found. In addition to producing auditory and visual hallucinations, these drugs produce a deep state of personal dissociation (i.e., an out-of-body experience), similar to that produced by meditation. This inhibits the recognition of being a person separate from one's surroundings and produces a sense of oneness with the universe that can be quite profound and life changing.

The three main drugs in this class are LSD, psilocybin, and DMT. LSD was synthesized in 1938 by Albert Hoffman. Hoffman synthesized LSD and other compounds from a group of natural compounds called ergot alkaloids that are found in rye fungus (see Figure 11.1A) while working for Sandoz Laboratories. Ergot alkaloids are natural compounds that contract smooth muscle and had been used for centuries to cause abortion,

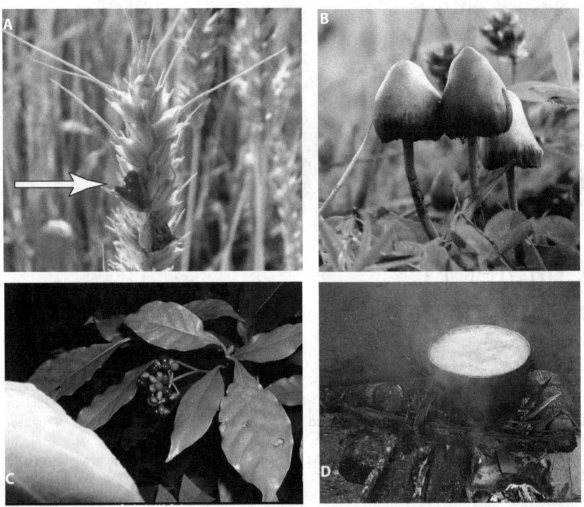

Figure 11.1 A. Ergot fungus growing on rye B. Psilocybe semilanceata mushrooms C. Psychotria viridis, a component of ayahuasca (Photo by Charles Bikle. © 2007 Erowid.org). D. Preparation of ayahuasca.

hasten childbirth, and slow excessive bleeding after childbirth. The compounds Hoffman synthesized turned out to be uninteresting for smooth-muscle pharmacology, so he put them in storage. Five years later, he retrieved LSD for other studies, accidentally ingested it, and discovered its psychedelic effects.

Psilocybin is a natural chemical derived from psilocybin mushrooms, also called magic mushrooms (see Figure 11.1B). There are several different genera of mushrooms that produce psilocybin, including *Psylocybe*, *Panaeolos*, and

Conocybe. Psilocybin is a very polar compound that is rapidly metabolized by the liver into psilocin, which is the psychoactive form of the drug.

DMT is also a natural chemical found in many plant and some animal species (there is some evidence that it is produced in the human brain). It has the same effects as LSD and psilocybin, but is metabolized very rapidly. Indigenous people of the Amazon basin combine DMT-containing plants (e.g., *Psychotria viridis*; see Figure 11.1C) with a vine that has a chemical that inhibits DMT metabolism (*Banisteriopsis caapi*) to produce ayahuasca (see Figure 11.1D).

Pharmacokinetics

All of these drugs produce the same effects by activating serotonin receptors (see Figure 11.2). The main difference among them is their pharmacokinetics. LSD and psilocybin are typically consumed orally. LSD is the most potent of the drugs, with a dose range of 25 to 500 micrograms, with a typical dose being 100 micrograms. This amount is so small that it is usually dissolved in a solvent and blotted onto paper for use (see Figure 11.3). Psilocybin, usually taken in the form of dried mushrooms, is less potent; a typical dose of psilocybin is 10 to 20 milligrams. DMT is usually snorted or smoked (due to its active first-pass metabolism). A DMT dose is slightly higher than psilocybin, 20 to 50 milligrams.

LSD and psilocybin are similar in their time to peak and duration of action. Effects of LSD can be felt in thirty to ninety minutes and peak in three hours. It can then last six to twelve hours after peak. The effects of psilocybin begin approximately one hour after oral administration and peak in two hours. Psilocybin lasts six to ten hours after peak. DMT is very different from these two, peaking in as little as five minutes

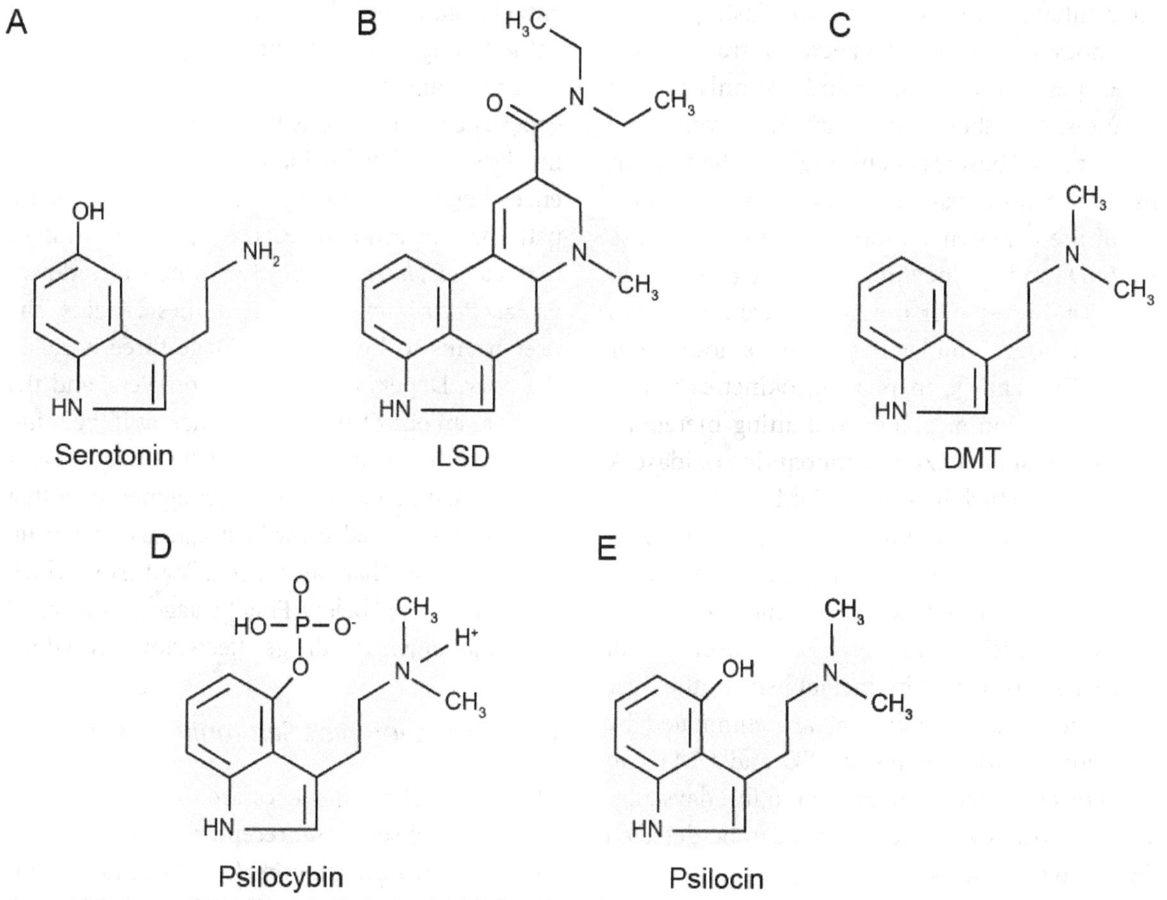

Figure 11.2 Areas of structural similarity are highlighted in yellow.

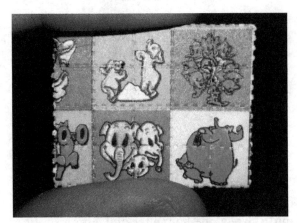

Figure 11.3 Because of its extremely high potency, a very low dose is taken. For this reason, LSD is typically dissolved in a solvent and blotted on paper for distribution.

after inhalation or snorting and lasting up to one hour after peak. If injected intravenously, it can peak in one minute and last only twenty minutes. This short time course has given it the slang term "businessman's high." When taken in the form of ayahuasca, the pharmacokinetics of the experience more closely follow those of LSD and psilocybin, beginning thirty to ninety minutes after ingestion, peaking in two to three hours, and lasting up to six hours after peak. This change in pharmacokinetics is due to the addition of plants containing metabolic inhibitors of the enzyme monoamine oxidase A (MAO-A), which inactivates DMT.

LSD and DMT are nonpolar and easily cross the blood-brain barrier. Psilocybin, as mentioned above, is polar but is rapidly metabolized to psilocin, which is nonpolar. The effects of all three are terminated by metabolism in the liver to inactive compounds that are eliminated by the kidneys. Metabolites of LSD and DMT can be detected in the urine for two to five days after use, and psilocybin metabolites can be detected for up to seven days.

The Psychedelic Experience

The psychedelic experience, often called a "trip," is an altered psychological state with profound hallucinations, sometimes referred to as *induced psychosis*. The visual hallucinations include some or all of the following: colors change and become more vibrant; shapes of people and objects distort and expand; geometric shapes appear; the ordinary sense of time passing disappears; or synesthesia, the crossover of senses (seeing sounds, hearing colors, etc.) occurs. Cognitive changes include profound depersonalization, as if standing outside the self and watching, and spiritual awakening or merging with the universe. The last aspect, spiritual awakening, is why these drugs are considered to be entheogenic. The user enters a state resembling religious ecstasy that is enlightening and can be life changing.

There are four stages to the psychedelic experience. Stage one is the *onset*. This primarily involves visual hallucinations. The user experiences heightened, exaggerated senses; geometric patterns appear, and objects change shape. In stage two, called *plateau*, subjective time slows down, visual effects intensify, and synesthesia begins. The user begins to lose control. Stage three is called the *peak*. Depersonalization is complete, and the user has an out-of-body experience, as if the mind is in another world. This usually includes self-reflection, understanding, and enlightenment that can cause personal growth. It can also bring up bad memories that can cause a "bad trip," which will be discussed below. Finally, stage four is called the *come-down*. The drug's effects slowly recede.

Pharmacodynamics: Serotonin Receptors

The effects of psychedelics are due to activation of a subset of serotonin receptors. Serotonin, also called 5-hydroxytryptamine (5-HT), has seven different types of receptors (5-HT_1 through 5-HT_7), many of which have subtypes (5-HT$_{1A}$, 5-HT$_{1B}$, etc.), for a total of fourteen different receptors. All except the 5-HT$_3$ receptor are metabotropic, linking to their effects via G-proteins. The most prominent and widely studied serotonin receptors are the 5-HT1$_A$ and 5-HT$_{2A}$ receptors. Psychedelic drugs are mainly agonists of the 5-HT$_{2A}$ receptors.

5-HT$_{2A}$ receptors are concentrated in the cortex and are also found in the thalamus, hippocampus, cerebellum, brain stem, and spinal cord (see Figure 8.7 for spinal cord location and function). These receptors are found both pre- and postsynaptically in synapses in the cortex. The second messenger system they use, not discussed previously, involves the activation of phospholipase C (PLC). PLC produces diacylglycerol (DAG), which activates protein kinase C (PKC). PKC phosphorylates calcium channels, leading to an increased entry of Ca^{2+} (see Figure 11.4). The increased Ca^{2+} increases glutamate release from the presynaptic axon bulb and increases the EPSPs evoked by the glutamate postsynaptically. Overstimulation of glutamate signaling by psychedelics results in dramatic increases in spontaneous EPSPs in the postsynaptic neurons, which disrupts normal functioning in the brain and produces self-generated thoughts and sensory experiences.

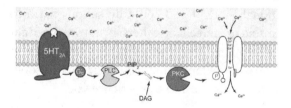

Figure 11.4 5-HT2a receptors on presynaptic axon bulbs of glutamate neurons activate a G-protein that activates Phospholipase C (PLC). PLC breaks down a phospholipid (PIP2) to release diacylglycerol (DAG) that, in turn, activates Proteins Kinase C (PKC). PKC uses ATP to phosphorylate voltage dependent calcium channels, causing them to stay open longer and admit more Ca^{2+}, resulting in more glutamate release.

Pharmacodynamics: Pathways and Effects

One effect of psychedelic drugs is the disinhibition of the normal thalamic-cortex connection. They block the filtering function of the thalamus, which normally lets only important information come to conscious awareness, and floods the PCF with sensory information unscreened. Another effect is the hyperstimulation of the visual sensory regions in the occipital lobes (by increasing glutamate release) and increased connectivity of this lobe to other sensory regions (the parietal and temporal lobes). The combination of the hyperstimulation and loss of filtering function produces hallucinations. These are self-generated images and patterns (often geometric) produced by the visual cortex as if it were receiving input, although it is not (see Figure 11.5). The increased connectivity between the visual and other sensory regions produces synesthesia. This is a crossing over of senses: sounds (especially music) are associated with specific colors, shapes, or other sounds; visuals can be felt or spontaneous visuals can be seen; colors and sounds have a taste or smell; and so on. The hallucinations can involve

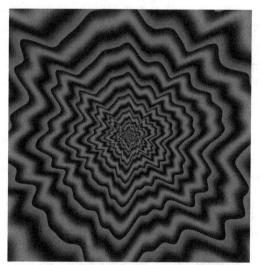

Figure 11.5 This is a geometric pattern suggestive of the visual hallucinations produced by psychedelic drugs.

the distortion of actual people or objects or the creation of entirely fictitious ones.

The effects on cognition are separate from the hallucinations and more important both recreationally and therapeutically (see Box 11.1). The major fMRI findings with psychedelics indicate that there is a dramatic blockage of the default-mode network (DMN). Regions of the DMN especially affected are in the posterior of the brain: the posterior cingulate cortex (PCC), lateral parietal lobe (LPL), and precuneus. These posterior regions normally create a sense of self (i.e., who and where I am right now in time) and communicate this to the medial prefrontal cortex (MPC) of the DMN. These regions become disconnected from the executive functions of the MPC, resulting in ego-dissolution or depersonalization. This is the source of the out-of-body experience. The self is no longer distinguished from its surroundings. The person becomes one with the outside world.

This depersonalization and oneness is the key to the spiritual or entheogenic properties of psychedelics. Ego-dissolution is accompanied by an altered sense of meaning in the surroundings. Unimportant things take on new, alien, and salient meanings. These experiences are described as transcendent, mystical experiences; users describe a feeling of being at one with the universe or "encountering God." It is likened to the state of bliss achieved by long-time meditators in a trance. Indeed, fMRI studies of meditators show similar changes in DMN activity as those of subjects tested with psychedelics. This experience can produce long-lasting changes in the user's personality. Some users consider their "trip" as among the most significant experiences of their lives and derive personal growth from it.

Thus, the main effects of psychedelics can be attributed to overstimulation of specific glutamate pathways that creates spontaneous activity and opens neural pathways. Visual effects spontaneously generated in the occipital lobes are combined with senses from the other lobes of the cerebral cortex and allowed to pass unfiltered through the thalamus to the MPC. The MPC is disconnected from other nodes in the DMN, creating a feeling of spiritual oneness with the world, which can cause profound and long-lasting changes in a person's personality.

Negative Effects

Psychedelics such as LSD are nearly impossible to overdose on in the classical sense (see Figure 10.10). The receptors for these drugs are in regions of the brain that are not necessary for minute-to-minute maintenance for life support as are, for example, opiate receptors. The addiction potential of hallucinogens is also very low. They don't directly or indirectly affect dopamine in the limbic system, which is the center of addiction in the brain. Also, 5-HT_{2A} receptors downregulate with repeated psychedelic use; the effects of the drugs quickly diminish.

However, hallucinations can lead one to do unpredictable, dangerous things. The classic saying in the 1960s was, "I'm not going to jump; I'm going to fly!" The user is disconnected from rational thought and could do serious harm to himself or herself or others if not in the right environment. This is why it is important to be in a safe place when taking these drugs with a sober guide to help make the experience safe.

Another danger with these drugs is the possibility of a "bad trip." This is a nightmarish experience that can include paranoia, panic, and extreme delusions. It can be caused by the user fearing the loss of control or by bringing up repressed memories of traumatic events. It can also be caused by an unsafe environment that triggers fear in the user. The effects will wear off

Major depression is an extremely debilitating disorder. Its symptoms are fatigue, a lack of self-worth, a loss of interest in life, anhedonia, insomnia, and overall feelings of sadness and worthlessness. It is a paralyzing condition that can lead to suicide. As discussed in Chapter 6, depression is characterized by excessive rumination on negative, self-referential thoughts. Self-referential thinking is a process of the DMN, and, not surprisingly, fMRI studies show decreased activity in the anterior cingulate cortex (ACC, part of the salience network, SN) and dorsolateral prefrontal cortex (DLPC, part of the task-positive network, TPN). Also, there is overactivity of the connections between the medial prefrontal cortex (MPC, part of the DMN) and the amygdala, the emotion center of the limbic system. The SN is unable to direct attention away from the DMN to the TPN due to chronic underactivity of the ACC, and the person becomes trapped in emotionally damaging self-reflection.

The connections between the different centers in the brain are mainly under the control of glutamate and GABA neurons. Other neurotransmitters, specifically serotonin, norepinephrine, and dopamine, modulate the activity of glutamate and GABA neurons, tweaking their release up and down. Serotonin, as discussed in the text, increases the release of glutamate. Therefore, drugs that modify serotonin levels, particularly selective serotonin reuptake inhibitors (SSRIs), can be effective in treating people with depression. However, up to 20% of people with major depression are resistant to all of the pharmacological treatments currently employed.

Recent research suggests that hallucinogens may be useful in treating these drug-resistant forms of major depression. Ketamine has received the most attention, probably because it is listed as a Schedule II drug by the DEA and is available to physicians and researchers. Ketamine blocks NMDA receptors, disrupting the connectivity in all pathways in the brain, including the DMN. In addition to disruption of the destructive DMN pathways, ketamine is associated with stimulating activity in the ACC, potentially increasing SN activity. When given in sub-anesthetic doses, it has been shown to produce mild dissociation that is correlated with rapid alleviation of up to 50% of symptoms in many subjects. This relief is maximal twenty-four hours after the treatment and lasts up to a week. Unfortunately, the effect slowly wanes as the week goes on. This suggests that ketamine therapy would require weekly treatments, and, because the safety of prolonged usage is unclear, it may be of limited use.

Psychedelic hallucinogens such as LSD, psilocybin, and DMT have also been used in experimental studies of depression. As discussed in this chapter, these drugs directly activate 5-HT_{2A} receptors. One effect of this is to block the posterior areas of the DMN (posterior cingulate cortex, lateral parietal lobe, and precuneus), which are responsible for the generation of the self-awareness. This causes depersonalization. The hope is that in a therapeutic environment, the disintegrated self can be redirected away from negative and into to positive thought patterns. In addition, 5-HT_{2A} receptors are highly expressed in the amygdala and ACC. Activation of these receptors by LSD or psilocybin may help break this overactive connection.

Studies have tested using psychedelics in terminal cancer patients experiencing anxiety and depression due to their diagnosis. The results show that more than half of participants showed significant improvement in symptoms, which allowed them to enjoy the time they had left. The most interesting aspect of these studies was that a single psychedelic experience produced changes that lasted months to years after one session. Similar experiments were done with volunteers with obsessive compulsive disorder, alcoholism, and nicotine addiction with similar success rates and durations. The extraordinary duration of a single dose of these drugs may be due to a hyper-release of glutamate, which could be activating neuroadaptation or neurotoxicity, cementing the changes. It could also be that the salience of the experience increases its long-term impact. However, the reason for its lasting impact is speculation, and much more research needs to be done.

While the studies of psychedelics are promising, it is important to note that these studies are in their infancy. Few studies have yet been done, and those that have been conducted have included small numbers of test subjects. However, the relatively safety of these drugs when used in the context of a therapeutic relationship suggest that this may be an important future area of psychiatric study.

in time and can be mitigated by anxiolytics (e.g., Valium) or often by "talking down" the panicky user. The danger of a bad trip is another good reason to have a sober guide.

Finally, there have been cases of a psychedelic experience precipitating latent psychosis. As discussed in Chapter 10, schizophrenia is a result of over-pruning of axon bulbs in the cortex (See Figure 10.11). One of the things that can cause axon loss is excitotoxicity; an extreme release of glutamate overstimulates cells, causing an increase of internal Ca^{2+}, which leads to apoptosis of the nerve cell. Psychedelics increase glutamate release, producing hyperexcitability; this may be the mechanism of the precipitation of psychosis. However, it should be noted that this is only seen in people who are already predisposed to schizophrenia for genetic or developmental reasons.

Flashbacks and HPPD

A *flashback* is a recurrence of the psychedelic experience days, weeks, or years after abstinence from the drug. They are usually short, spontaneous (with no specific trigger), and reversible. The main effect is visual hallucination, although auditory hallucination can also occur.

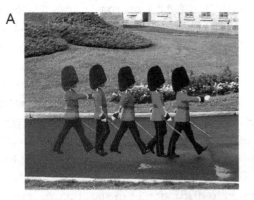

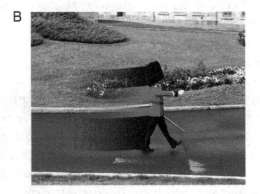

Figure 11.6 A. Trailing images are when a moving object has a series of static images of the object following in its path. B. Afterimages are when a continuous blur of the image trails behind its movement.

Salvia divinorum (salvia) is a plant native to the Oaxaca region of Mexico. Like psilocybin mushrooms, it has been used in religious rituals by indigenous people for centuries. Knowledge of this plant has become more widespread recently because of its recreational use. It has not been made illegal federally in the United States; however, several states have banned its sale and use.

Its active ingredient, salvinorum A, is the most potent natural hallucinogen known, in the range of potency of LSD (10- to 500-microgram doses). Leaves of the plant are usually smoked or chewed (for oral absorption), as salvinorum A is inactivated in the digestive tract. Salvia produces an intense, brief hallucinogenic experience, similar to that of the serotoninergic hallucinogens. A typical salvia trip can last from ten to fifteen minutes to an hour.

What is most curious about salvia is its mechanism of action. Salvinorum A is an agonist of κ-opioid receptors. These receptors are typically activated by dynorphin and produce dysphoria in the nucleus accumbens. However, κ-opioid receptors are also widely distributed in the cerebral cortex. The salvia trip includes visual hallucinations, depersonalization, recalling past events and a profound entheogenic sensation. Thus, the effects of this drug are very similar to activation of 5-HT_{2A} receptors, despite the fact that the drug has no activity at these receptors at all.

The hallucinations can be geometric patterns, changing colors, shapes moving and changing, afterimages, trailing images, and other visual disturbances usually seen during onset stage of the psychedelic experience (see Figure 11.6). These can range from pleasant to disturbing, depending on the person experiencing them and his or her past experiences with psychedelics.

Hallucinogen persisting perception disorder (HPPD) is a condition similar to flashbacks, except that it is more subtle and persistent. HPPD occurs in a minority of psychedelic users (1 to 5%) and is initiated and intensified by chronic, repeated use. People with HPPD see subtle light halos around people and objects, trailing images, afterimages behind moving objects, colors changing or intensifying, and objects changing in size and distorting in shape. They also tend to be more aware of normal visual distortions, such as floaters in the eyes and white spots cause by blood cells in the retina. This can be distressing to the person because of the chronic, irreversible nature of the effects.

The causes of flashbacks and HPPD are still unknown, although the common idea that the drug is stored in the fat or spinal cord and later released is apocryphal. One hypothesis is that the drugs induce the expression of metabolic enzymes (e.g., catecholamine O-methyl transferase) that disrupt the balance between catecholamines (norepinephrine and dopamine) and serotonin. New evidence that SSRIs can precipitate flashbacks suggests that the psychedelic experience causes changes in the visual system (possibly through neuroadaptation) that make users more susceptible to hallucinations when serotonin levels are high. 5-HT2 receptors are found on both excitatory (glutamate) and inhibitory (GABA) neurons in the primary visual cortex of the occipital lobe. Decreasing inhibitory input or increasing excitatory input can create afterimages. Increasing both can create trailing images. This suggests that neuroadaptation in GABA and glutamate neurons may be involved in these phenomena.

Dissociative Hallucinogens

History

Dissociative hallucinogens are synthetic drugs that were developed as anesthetic drugs in the 1950s and '60s. The goal was to produce a drug that had the desired qualities of anesthetics (to produce unconsciousness, amnesia, and analgesia) without the respiratory depression produced by the barbiturates that were currently in use. The first drug developed was phencyclidine (PCP, or angel dust; see Figure 11.7A). This drug seemed promising at first, as it produced profound anesthesia, amnesia, and analgesia. However, the anesthesia produced was likened to a catatonic psychotic state (stiff, rigid body), as opposed to the relaxed anesthesia desired. In addition, patients waking after PCP anesthesia were often agitated and confused, sometimes violent, and would often experience hallucinations and distressing delusions. For these reasons,

clinical use of PCP was discontinued, although it is still sometimes used as an animal tranquilizer. Recreational use of the drug began in the late 1960s and grew through the '70s, but tapered off because of the ill effects it produced and the stigma attached to its use.

Ketamine synthesis followed that of PCP, and its clinical use began in the 1960s (see Figure 11.7B). This drug was more useful than PCP in that it did not produce agitation; however, disturbing hallucinations persisted and limited its use. It fell out of favor for years but has seen a resurgence of use recently. It has a shorter half-life than PCP (see below) and is used for brief, painful procedures, such as setting broken bones. It is particularly useful for opioid addicts, as opioids are no longer useful for pain relief or sedation in these patients. It is commonly used in veterinary medicine.

Dextromethorphan (DXM; see Figure 11.7C) was synthesized from an opioid precursor in the 1940s as a replacement for codeine for cough

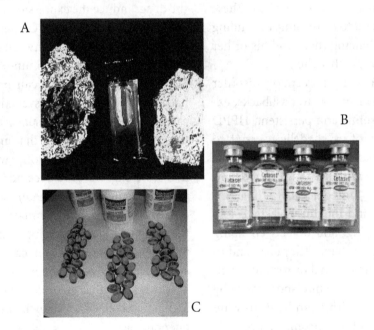

Figure 11.7 A. Phencyclidine (PCP) B. Ketamine C. Dextromethorphan (in the form of Robotussin pills)

suppression. Romilar, the first marketed version of DXM, was in tablet form. This was soon discontinued because it was found that high doses induced hallucinations and depersonalization; recreational use in this form exceeded its intended use. DXM was then formulated into syrups (e.g., Robitussin DM, thus the term "Robo rolling"), with the thought that the syrup would discourage recreational use. However, cough syrup is still abused for its hallucinogenic properties.

These three drugs have multiple effects, and experiences with each are different. However, they share a common dissociative and hallucinogenic mechanism and are categorized together for this reason.

Pharmacokinetics

There are many differences among these three drugs based on their pharmacokinetics. PCP is usually smoked by dissolving it in a solvent and then either spraying it on plant material (e.g., oregano or mint) or using the solution to saturate a tobacco or cannabis cigarette. It is also taken orally or injected, and can be snorted if obtained in a pure enough form. A typical dose is from 3 to 10 milligrams. When smoked, injected, or snorted, the effects come on rapidly, producing a rush of euphoria, and diminish in four to six hours. When orally consumed, effects begin in thirty to sixty minutes and last five to eight hours. It is inactivated by metabolism in the liver, and the metabolic products are excreted by the kidneys. PCP is nonpolar and concentrates in fatty tissues; for this reason, its effects linger as long as twenty-four hours, and it can be detected in the urine for up to a week after use.

Ketamine is difficult to synthesize in clandestine labs, so it is usually stolen from pharmacies or veterinary offices in sterile vials dissolved in saline. It can be either injected or ingested in this form or dried to powder and snorted. A low to moderate dose is 30 to 50 milligrams; a high dose is typically 60 to 250 milligrams, depending on the route of administration. Bioavailability is about 50% via nasal route and 20% via oral administration (due to significant first-pass metabolism), which is why larger doses are taken orally. Effects begin within minutes of injection or snorting and after thirty minutes following oral administration. Ketamine has a relatively short duration of action, lasting from thirty to forty-five minutes via injection, forty-five to sixty minutes for snorting, and one to two hours after oral administration. Ketamine can be detected in the urine two to four days after use, and its metabolites can be detected seven to fourteen days after use.

DXM is usually consumed orally in the form of cough syrup. The antitussive dose is 20 to 30 milligrams, while the recreational dose can vary from 100 milligrams to 1,500 milligrams, depending on the depth of the experience sought. It is metabolized in the liver during the first pass; this metabolism is greatly affected by genetics and varies considerably between users. DXM is metabolized to dextrorphan on first pass, which is also psychoactive and produces the same effects. The effects can take a long time to peak, especially for high doses. Time to onset of effect is from thirty to ninety minutes; peak effects can take up to three hours and can last three to six hours after peak. DXM and its metabolites are usually not tested for in the urine because DXM is legal. However, DXM can often produce false positives in urine tests for opioids or PCP, depending on the dose and the length of time since it was taken.

Pharmacodynamics

These drugs are what pharmacologists call "dirty" drugs. This means that although they were designed to affect one receptor and produce one effect, they actually affect many different receptors. They usually have the highest affinity for the receptor that is being targeted (and therefore affect it at low doses) and begin to activate other receptors at higher doses, changing the effect. For example, while ketamine produces its main effects by blocking the N-methyl-D-aspartate (NMDA) receptor (see below), it also blocks the nicotinic and muscarinic acetylcholine receptors, activates dopamine receptors, inhibits the uptake pumps for serotonin, dopamine, and norepinephrine, and blocks calcium channels, in addition to other mechanisms; each of these mechanisms has a different dose range.

The main mechanism of these drugs, and the one that they have in common, is blocking one of the receptors for glutamate. As discussed in Chapter 3, glutamate is an excitatory neurotransmitter. It has two receptors that are distinguished by drugs that specifically activate each one: the NMDA receptor and the α-amino-3-hydroxy-5-methyl-4-isoxazolepropionic acid receptor (AMPA receptor). These are both ionotropic receptors that pass cations (mostly Na^+) and produce EPSPs. NMDA receptors are the main receptors used during neurotransmission. AMPA receptors are found in the same synapses as NMDA receptors; they are involved in synaptic plasticity of highly active synapses. NMDA receptors are responsible for most of the excitatory activity in the brain and are found in every part of it. Partially blocking NMDA receptors decreases neurotransmission in these synapses, and totally blocking them shuts off neurotransmission.

The main effect seen recreationally from these drugs is dissociation, or depersonalization;

this is similar to the out-of-body experience described above for psychedelic hallucinogens. It is most likely due to segregating the nodes of the DMN, that is, separating the parts of the brain involved with the sense of self (precuneus and LPL) from the executive functions of the MPC, as happens with psychedelics. However, unlike psychedelics, the depersonalization is not accompanied by spiritual awakening or growth-inducing self-reflection. NMDA receptors are important for memory, including working memory (in the DLPC), episodic memory (in the hippocampus), and long-term memory (in the association areas of the cortex). As a result, these drugs all produce amnesia. PCP and ketamine also directly activate dopamine receptors in the same dose range as NMDA receptors, producing mild to moderate euphoria. This makes them the only addictive hallucinogenic drugs.

Higher doses of these drugs produce a more intense experience. As dose increases, PCP produces numbness to a complete block of feeling in the extremities (analgesia), due to blockage of NMDA receptors and activation of opioid receptors. NMDA-receptor blockage produces profound depersonalization at high doses and also PFC stimulation, which can lead to aggression and paranoid ideation and/or detachment from the physical surroundings. Visual and auditory hallucinations also appear at these doses, as well as amnesia. This can produce a person who is irate, insensitive to physical stimuli, and out of their mind, similar to what happens during a psychotic episode. Although this is a less frequent occurrence than suggested in the media, it presents a very difficult situation for law enforcement: a raging individual entirely insensitive to pain. At even higher doses, PCP produces anesthesia, catatonia, convulsions, and respiratory depression, which can cause death.

At high doses, ketamine activates 5-HT receptors, blocks muscarinic receptors (discussed below in the section on deliriants), and activates μ- and κ-opioid receptors. This produces visual hallucinations, auditory hallucinations, and analgesia in addition to the depersonalization and amnesia caused by blocking NMDA receptors. This is called "going down the K-hole." The user experiences profound detachment from the body and the world, moderate euphoria, loss of time perception, and visual and auditory hallucinations. The user has a sense of floating in another world, detached from the real world. Activation of κ-opioid receptors can produce dysphoria in some users.

DXM and its metabolic product dextrorphan affect many receptors in addition to blocking NMDA receptors. They produce a high-affinity block of both the serotonin and norepinephrine reuptake pumps. They also have high affinity at μ-and κ-opioid receptors, like ketamine does. However, the relative action at each of these sites is apparently different because the effects of high dose DXM are distinctly different from those of PCP or ketamine. DXM produces dissociation, due to the NMDA receptor block, but produces more stimulation, possibly by blocking norepinephrine reuptake. Hallucinations tend to appear as visual distortions, rather than full-blown patterns and shapes. Similar to PCP and ketamine, it causes a loss of the sense of time passing.

In general, these three drugs are grouped together because of their common blockade of NMDA receptors, which produces depersonalization and loss of the sense of time by blocking the DMN connections between the front and rear of the brain. They produce euphoria, either by blocking dopamine reuptake or direct action on dopamine receptors. And they produce amnesia by blocking NMDA receptors in the hippocampus and DLPC. However, they each produce other effects due to the many different receptor sites that each drug can affect. These receptor sites vary based on the particular drug's affinity for each, which causes additional hallucinatory, analgesic, euphoric, and emotional effects that vary by drug.

Negative Effects

Despite frequent negative effects (dysphoria and disturbing hallucinations), these drugs produce euphoria, especially early in the experience, and for this reason are addictive and have serious long-term effects. Studies in chronic users have shown decreases in gray and white matter in prefrontal cortex regions involved in TPN and DMN functioning. As such, these users have impaired executive abilities, which make it difficult to focus on a task or make decisions. They also have impaired memory function. Depression is common in chronic users, as are schizophrenic-like symptoms and flashbacks.

Deliriant Hallucinogens

History

Delirium is a state of mental confusion. It represents a loss of control of the normal cognitive networks (TPN, DMN, and SN), resulting in an inability to focus or perform meaningful activities. It can be accompanied by excitement or sedation. When produced by deliriant hallucinogens, it includes vivid visual hallucinations.

Deliriant hallucinogens have been common in medicinal, religious, and shamanistic practices for centuries. They are natural products that are found in members of a family of plants called the nightshades (*Solanaceae*), which are found all around the world. This family includes the plants jimsonweed (*Datura*), deadly nightshade (belladonna), stinking nightshade (henbane), and mandrake root (see Figure 11.8).

These plants all produce compounds called *tropane alkaloids*, which include the drugs atropine and scopolamine. Traditionally, preparations of these plants were used as analgesics, as anesthetics, and for asthma. They were also commonly used as poisons, because high doses are lethal. Like most hallucinogens, they were also used in spiritual practices to produce visions and a sensation of taking flight. Atropine and scopolamine are still used in medicinal applications today. The most common use of atropine is in ophthalmic examinations, blocking muscarinic receptors to cause extreme widening of the pupils for examination of the retina. Scopolamine is used in transdermal patches for motion sickness.

Pharmacokinetics

Jimsonweed is a small flowering plant with leaves similar to the dandelion that is native to

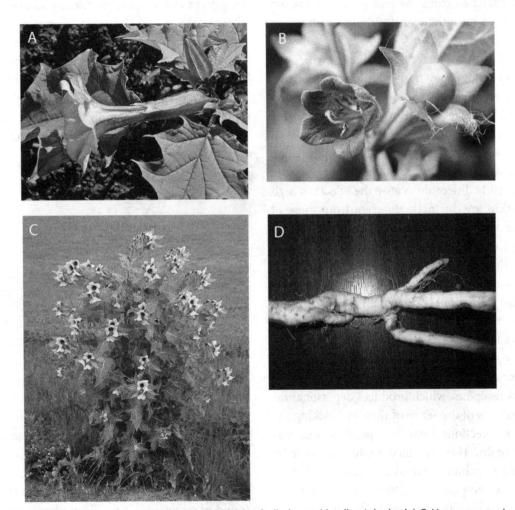

Figure 11.8 A. Datura stramonium (Jimson weed) B. Atropa belladonna (deadly nightshade) C. Hyoscyamus niger (henbane) D. Mandragora officinarum (mandrake root).

North America. The leaves and seeds can be eaten or smoked. The seeds of the belladonna and henbane plants have been used in tinctures (alcohol extracts) or decoctions (boiled in water). Mandrake root is usually dried and crushed into a power that is added to water or wine. Absorption depends on the route of administration; it is rapid for smoked plants and slower for oral administration.

Atropine and scopolamine are both somewhat nonpolar, and both easily cross all biological barriers. Atropine is only partially metabolized in the liver; approximately 50% is excreted unchanged. A typical dose can last from two to four hours. Scopolamine is actively metabolized in the liver and not very effective in oral administration. It has a short half-life and is typically delivered in a transdermal patch to achieve a constant dose for as long as the patch is adhered (up to three days).

Mechanism of Action

Atropine and scopolamine are muscarinic receptor antagonists. Muscarinic receptors are metabotropic receptors that are linked through different G-protein isoforms to produce (1) inhibition of cyclic AMP formation, (2) activation of K^+ channels, or (3) activation of phospholipase C and increased Ca^{2+} entry (as in 5-HT_{2A} receptors above; see Figure 11.4). The mechanism used depends on the location of the receptor and the G-protein isoform found there.

Muscarinic receptors are found in both the peripheral and central nervous systems. In the peripheral nervous system, they are the receptors used by the parasympathetic nervous system. This is the "rest-and-digest" system discussed briefly in Chapter 4. Activating the muscarinic receptors of the parasympathetic system causes a decrease in heat rate, increased salivation, increased gastric and intestinal motility, bladder contraction and urination, tear formation, sexual arousal, and sweating. Sweat glands are one rare instance of muscarinic receptors in the sympathetic nervous system (which usually releases norepinephrine). Sweat is produced by sympathetic neurons that release acetylcholine onto muscarinic receptors. Blocking peripheral muscarinic receptors with atropine or scopolamine produces uncomfortable side effects: rapid heart rate, constipation, difficulty urinating, dry eyes, dry mouth, and hot, dry skin.

Muscarinic receptors are found in many places in the brain, with concentrations in the brain stem/midbrain (RAS), striatum (nucleus accumbens and dorsal striatum), PFC, and visual cortex (occipital lobe). Blocking the muscarinic receptors in the RAS produces drowsiness/sedation. (One of the side effects of antihistamine drugs, such as diphenhydramine, is to produce sedation by blocking these muscarinic receptors.) This is why these drugs were traditionally used as anesthetics.

The deliriant effects of anti-muscarinics are due to effects in the visual cortex, PFC, and striatum. Inhibition of the association processing in the PFC causes a clouding of consciousness, making it difficult to think and focus on a task. Inhibition of the inhibitory role of muscarinic receptors in the occipital (visual) cortex results in increased stimulation, resulting in spontaneous visual stimulation and hallucinations.

An interesting hypothesis of the deliriant effects of these drugs involves the role of the thalamus as a filtering center of the brain (see Figure 11.9A). The thalamus receives all incoming sensory information and filters it to determine which inputs are most important. These sensory signals are sent to the cortex for processing and conscious awareness. GABAergic neurons from the striatum (part of the limbic system) innervate the thalamus

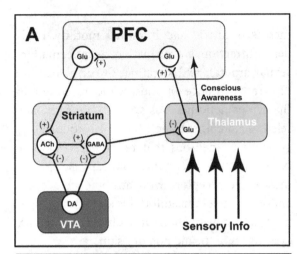

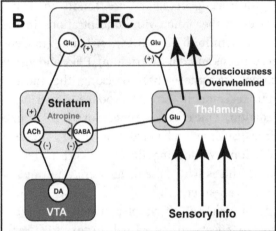

Figure 11.9 A. Under normal circumstances, GABAergic neurons from the striatum inhibit the thalamus; this increases its filtering of sensory information. This inhibition is augmented by acetylcholine (ACh) being released by other interneurons in the striatum, which is stimulate by feedback neurons from the prefrontal cortex (PFC). As a result, is only important sensory information reaching conscious awareness. Dopamine released by the ventral tegmental area (VTA) inhibits this loop and decreases filtering. B. Anti-muscarinic drugs, like atropine, block the effect of ACh on the GABAergic neurons. The result is less GABA inhibition on the thalamus, less thalamic screening, and more sensory information reaching conscious awareness unfiltered.

as part of this filtering process. GABA in the thalamus increases its filtering of sensory information. Acetylcholine-releasing neurons in the striatum stimulate these GABA neurons and inhibit the thalamus when nothing important is going on (imagine driving down a highway, not paying much attention to the scenery). When something important happens that requires attention (e.g., a car pulling into your lane), the ventral tegmental area (VTA) releases dopamine in the limbic system, including the acetylcholine neurons and GABA neurons, inhibiting both. The inhibition of these neurons stops their inhibition of the thalamus, allowing more sensory information to pass through the thalamus to the cerebral cortex; you suddenly become aware of your surroundings and focus in order to address the situation. A glutamate feedback loop from the PFC to the striatum activates the acetylcholine neurons to inhibit the thalamus; this feedback ensures that information from the thalamus doesn't overload the PFC's cognitive resources (i.e., its ability to deal with incoming information).

Anti-muscarinics decrease the thalamic-filtering process (see Figure 11.9B). They block the muscarinic receptors on the GABAergic neurons, stopping them from being stimulated in the striatum. By blocking the excitatory input on the GABAergic neurons, they become less active and release less inhibitory GABA in the thalamus. The thalamus stops screening sensory information, resulting in a flood of sensory input into the cortex; simultaneously, anti-muscarinics block the inhibitory feedback pathway from the PFC that should limit sensory overload. The flood of sensory information overwhelms the ability of the cortex (especially the PFC) to operate efficiently. The result is cognitive overload (delirium) and hallucinations.

Negative Effects

The use of deliriant hallucinogens is uncommon, but not because of the difficulty in obtaining them. Jimsonweed can be found growing wild, and other plant products with atropine and scopolamine are readily available. Their use is uncommon because the side effects are usually very uncomfortable and the hallucinations produced are disturbing. The peripheral side effects (cited above) can last for twenty-four to forty-eight hours in the case of orally consumed seeds, which will slowly break down and release atropine. High doses produce hot, dry, flushed skin, dizziness, headache, and vomiting. Higher doses cause respiratory depression and death. One of the dangers of these drugs, especially jimsonweed, is that the concentration of active chemicals can vary dramatically in the wild grown plant. This makes it difficult to determine a safe dose.

Stimulant Hallucinogens

History

This group of drugs is another offshoot of the chemosynthetic experiments of the early twentieth century. As with LSD and amphetamines, these compounds were synthesized based on the structures of chemicals that were known to activate norepinephrine receptors in a search for vasoactive compounds. The basic plan was to add functional groups to the structure of a chemical known to have interesting effects and see how these changes modified the activity of the compound. Also, analogous to LSD, when these compounds were found to be uninteresting as vasoactive compounds, they were shelved and forgotten for decades, only to be rediscovered in the mid-twentieth century in the search for psychoactive compounds.

In the early 1960s, the discovery that some of these drugs helped a person open up emotionally led them to be used in psychotherapy. Psychiatrists who had success using these drugs with their patients spread the practice to their colleagues by word of mouth. The interesting effects of the drugs, combined with the open, experimental attitudes of the times, lead to the drugs being synthesized for recreational use. Once recreational use became widespread, their synthesis and distribution were made illegal. However, each individual chemical structure must be legislated in order to make it illegal. The demand for these drugs spawned a market for "designer drugs." These are drugs that are similar in structure to the outlawed drugs, with slight chemical modifications, so that the compounds are no longer covered under existing laws. These are then sold openly, until the legal system catches up with them. (Designer drugs today are sold legally as "synthetic marijuana" and "bath salts.")

Chemicals in this group are an alphabet soup of letters: DOM, DOB, MDA, MDEA, MDMA, and MDMC are examples; their acronyms are based on their chemical structures. These compounds have similar effects based on activity at monoamine receptors (i.e., norepinephrine, dopamine, and serotonin receptors). The best known of this group, which will be used as the main example in this chapter, is 3,4-methylene-dioxymethamphetamine (MDMA), or ecstasy (see Figure 11.10A).

MDMA was synthesized in 1912 by Merck Pharmaceuticals. Its psychoactive effects were first studied by Alexander Shulgin in the mid-1970s. He helped spread its use in the psychotherapist community through the early 1980s, when it started seeing use as a street drug. With the much more restrictive attitudes toward recreational drugs in the mid-1980s, MDMA became classified as a Schedule I drug (with no accepted medical uses), against the strong objections of

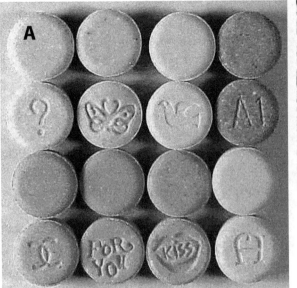
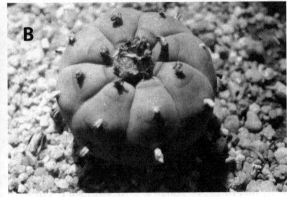

Figure 11.10 A. Ecstasy tablets. B. Lophophora williamsii (peyote cactus).

the psychotherapy community. However, due to MDMA's ease of synthesis and a stockpile of MDMA synthesized in the run-up to its outlaw, use of MDMA spread through the 1980s and into the 1990s. The happy, energetic effects of the drug led to the development of rave culture, a phenomenon of large, clandestine dance parties with repetitive electronic music.

The history of mescaline is very different, although it is included here because it has similar effects. Mescaline is derived from the small, spineless peyote cactus (*Lophophora williamsii*) indigenous to Mexico and southwest Texas (see Figure 11.10B). Native Americans in these regions have used peyote in spiritual and medicinal practices for thousands of years, and its use spread through other Native American tribes in the nineteenth century during a revival of native spirituality. The Native American Church is the only group legally allowed to use mescaline for religious practices, although peyote buttons can be bought illicitly and used recreationally.

Pharmacokinetics

MDMA and mescaline are both taken orally. MDMA peaks in the blood ninety minutes to two hours after ingestion, and mescaline peaks in approximately one hour. The long time to peak and uncertain nature of street MDMA often leads to re-dosing and overdose. A typical dose of MDMA is between 50 and 200 milligrams; the typical dosage of mescaline is between 200 and 400 milligrams. Both drugs are relatively nonpolar and easily cross the blood-brain barrier.

MDMA is metabolized by the liver to active (MDA) and inactive compounds. A typical experience lasts three to four hours after peak. Approximately 20% of the original dose will be excreted by the kidneys unchanged, the rest as metabolites. Mescaline is less readily metabolized by the liver. A typical experience will last ten hours, and up to 50% of the mescaline is excreted unchanged by the kidneys.

Pharmacodynamics: MDMA

MDMA and mescaline have effects on monoamines (norepinephrine, dopamine, and serotonin) due to their structural similarity to these neurotransmitters (see Figure 11.11). MDMA produces its effects by indirectly increasing synaptic serotonin, norepinephrine, and, to a lesser extent, dopamine. It does this by affecting the reuptake and vesicle pumps for these neurotransmitters by a number of mechanisms. First, MDMA has a higher affinity for the reuptake amine pump than the neurotransmitter does and outcompetes it for entry to the axon bulb (thus blocking reuptake of the neurotransmitter). Second, once inside the bulb, it inhibits the amine pump on storage vesicles, depleting them of neurotransmitters and increasing its concentration in the cytoplasm. Third, it activates the TARR1 receptor on the membrane of the axon bulbs in the same manner as amphetamines do (the TAAR1 receptor was discussed on Chapter 9; see Figure 9.8). TAAR1 stimulates the production of cAMP, which activates protein kinase A (PKA), and activation of protein kinase C (PKC; see Figure 11.4). PKA and PKC phosphorylate the amine pumps in the plasma membrane and on the vesicles, which makes them reverse direction. This causes the axon bulb to dump the neurotransmitter into the synapse. Finally, MDMA and its metabolite MDA have agonist effects on 5-HT_{2A} receptors, directly activating them. In general, the main effect of MDMA is to greatly increase the synaptic concentrations of serotonin and norepinephrine and slightly increase dopamine concentrations.

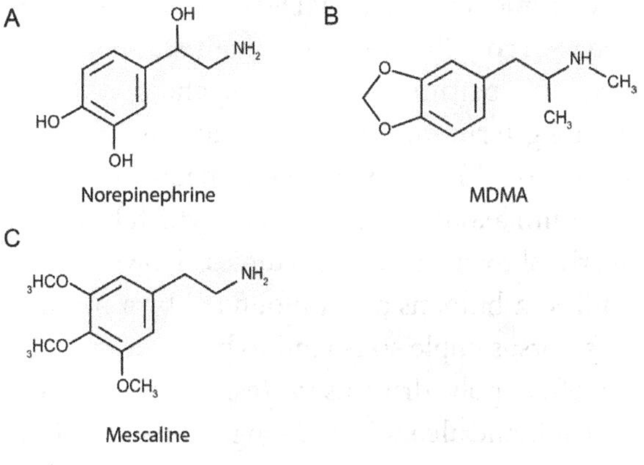

The effect of MDMA on mood and the production of visual hallucinations is due to the reversal of the serotonin reuptake pumps and activation of 5-HT_{2A} receptors (similar to LSD). This is dependent on the MDMA entering the axon bulb, and drugs that inhibit the reuptake pump (serotonin-selective reuptake inhibitors) block much of the MDMA effect. The other notable effect, stimulation, is due to the release of norepinephrine from axon terminals of the reticular activating system (RAS). MDMA is called a stimulant hallucinogen because of the combination of these two effects.

An important consequence of the increase of serotonin, rather than direct activation of 5-HT_{2A} receptors like LSD, is concurrent activation of 5-HT_{1A} receptors, which does not occur with LSD. 5-HT_{1A} and 5-HT_{2A} receptor activation cause the release of oxytocin in the brain and peripherally. Oxytocin is a peptide hormone produced in the hypothalamus. It is released into the bloodstream by the posterior pituitary and also into the nucleus accumbens (NA) of the limbic system. Oxytocin has many effects in the periphery, including uterine contraction during labor and milk letdown during lactation: Centrally, oxytocin promotes social bonding between mother and child and between intimate partners. The indirect release of oxytocin by MDMA makes it an empathogen/entactogen, increasing feelings of closeness between people; this is why it has been called the "love drug."

Figure 11.11 This is a structural comparison of A. norepinephrine, B. MDMA, and C. mescaline with the areas of structural similarity highlighted in yellow.

It creates feelings of empathy, opening people emotionally and causing interpersonal bonding.

The ecstasy experience is a combination of the effects of the oxytocin plus the three neurotransmitters it affects, with an emphasis on the serotonin and norepinephrine effects. Norepinephrine produces excitement and energy. Serotonin produces an overall sense of happiness and well-being, mild visual hallucinations (usually afterimages, as in Figure 11.6A), heightened pleasure in tactile sensory experiences, and loss of the sense of time passing. Oxytocin produces warm, close feelings of oneness with others. Mild dopamine release adds euphoria to the experience.

Pharmacodynamics: Mescaline

Mescaline, on the other hand, is an agonist at serotonin ($5\text{-}HT_{2A}$) and norepinephrine receptors and a partial agonist at dopamine receptors; it directly produces effects at these receptors. The mescaline experience typically begins with sympathomimetic effects (due to activity at peripheral norepinephrine receptors): rapid heart rate, increased blood pressure, sweating, and pupil dilation. Central norepinephrine receptors produce a sense of energy and loss of fatigue and appetite, similar to the effects of amphetamines. Central dopaminergic activity creates mild euphoria. Later, serotonergic effects begin. These are more typical of LSD than MDMA: altered sense of space and time, depersonalization, complex visual hallucinations (geometric patterns, color changes, people, animals), and synesthesia. In the third phase of the trip, mescaline is more like LSD than MDMA; it is entheogenic in this phase, creating a feeling of oneness with the universe. It is for this reason that mescaline is used in religious ceremonies of the Native American Church.

Negative Effects

While both MDMA and mescaline have dopaminergic effects, they tend not to be associated with addiction, as tolerance appears quickly. This is due to downregulation of receptors and, in the case of MDMA, depletion of serotonin in the nerve terminals. However, there is a serious risk of overdose with MDMA. One side effect of MDMA is hyperthermia. MDMA stimulates the hypothalamus to direct the parasympathetic nervous system to retain heat. It also produces dehydration; users at raves counter the dehydration with water, which can cause another problem, hyponatremia (low blood sodium). This occurs when the excess water is flushed out by the kidneys, along with too much sodium. In addition to hyperthermia, overdose with MDMA produces hypertension, hallucinations, disorientation, convulsions, coma, and death.

The flood of neurotransmitter release by MDMA causes serotonin depletion from these nerve terminals; the depletion can last from several days to two weeks after use. This causes a mild depression and fatigue, sometimes called "midweek blues." These effects decrease as levels of serotonin are reestablished in the nerve terminals.

Chronic, high-dose MDMA has been associated with cognitive deficits in many studies. These include impairments in working and short-term and long-term memory, as well as mild, chronic depression. This may be due to neurotoxicity in serotonin axons and axon bulbs, which has been clearly shown in animal studies. However, the studies in humans are confounded by a number of factors; sample sizes tend to be small, subjects are often poly drug users (especially co-using cannabis and alcohol), and longitudinal data (i.e., pre- and post-drug exposure testing) are lacking. Negative effects that are seen are, not surprisingly, correlated with size of dose, frequency of use, and duration of use.

Summary

There are four main classes of hallucinogens, based on their mechanism of action and effects. Psychedelics—represented by LSD, psilocybin, and DMT—are considered entheogenic for their ability to replicate mystical experiences. The psychedelic trip includes visual and auditory hallucinations, synesthesia, loss of the sense of time passing, depersonalization, and a sense of spiritual awakening. They produce this effect by activating the $5-HT_{2A}$ subtype of the serotonin receptor. This produces spontaneous EPSPs in the sensory cortex and an inhibition of the filtering function of the thalamus. The result is spontaneous signal generation and signal crossover in the sensory regions of the cortex, producing hallucinations and synesthesia. In addition, there is a shutdown of the posterior, ego-generating components of the DMN. This produces depersonalization, dissolution of the separation of the self from the environment, and a mystical experience.

Dissociative hallucinogens—PCP, ketamine, and DXM—were originally developed as anesthetic drugs. These drugs affect many receptors, but their main effect is to block NMDA receptors for glutamate. Because glutamate is the main excitatory neurotransmitter in the brain, high doses of these drugs produce anesthesia and amnesia. At lower doses, they can produce stimulation (resulting in hallucinations and unpredictable behavior) and the disconnection of the nodes of the DMN (producing depersonalization). However, the depersonalization produced by these drugs is not associated with a mystical experience, as with psychedelics. The production of mild euphoria makes these the only addictive hallucinogens.

Deliriant hallucinogens—mainly the anti-muscarinic drugs atropine and scopolamine—have been used for millennia in the Western tradition. They are usually used in their original plant form, that is, jimsonweed, deadly nightshade, henbane, and mandrake root, which contain atropine and scopolamine. These drugs block muscarinic acetylcholine receptors in the PFC, visual cortex, and striatum. This causes spontaneous visual stimulation and a blocking of the thalamic-filtering process (flooding the PFC with sensory info). The result is mental confusion and visual hallucinations.

Finally, stimulant hallucinogens (mescaline and MDMA) produce an excited hallucinogenic state. This is produced by mainly affecting norepinephrine and serotonin neurotransmission (with a mild effect on dopamine neurotransmission). These drugs differ in their mechanism of action; MDMA causes the release of serotonin and norepinephrine, while mescaline directly activates the receptors for these neurotransmitters. One consequence of the activation of all serotonin receptors (as opposed to only the $5-HT_{2A}$ receptors, as is the case with LSD) is the release of oxytocin. Oxytocin increases feelings of closeness and empathy between people, opens up people emotionally, and produces interpersonal bonding. This is unique to MDMA and why it is called the "love drug." Visual hallucinations caused by MDMA are minor and not considered important, while they are central to the effects of mescaline. Mescaline, which is a natural product used by people indigenous to Mexico and the southern United States, produces an amphetamine-like high that is later accompanied by an LSD-like trip. It is considered a spiritual experience, whereas the MDMA effect is not.

Further Reading

Indigenous use: Castaneda, Carlos. *The Teachings of Don Juan: A Yaqui Way of Knowledge.* Berkeley, CA: University of California Press, 1985.

Psychedelics: Nichols, David E. "Psychedelics." *Pharmacological Reviews* 68 (2016): 264–355.

Flashbacks: Litjensa, R. P.W., T. M. Bruntb, G. J. Alderliefstec, and R. H. S. Westerinka. "Hallucinogen Persisting Perception Disorder and the Serotonergic System: A Comprehensive Review, Including New MDMA-Related Clinical Cases." *European Neuropsychopharmacology* 24 (2014): 1309–23.

Psilocybin fMRI: Carhart-Harris, R. L., D. Erritzoe, T. Williams, J. M. Stone, L. J. Reeda, A. Colasantia, R. J. Tyackea, R. Leech, A. L. Maliziab, K. Murphy, P. Hobden, J. Evans, A. Feilding, R. G. Wise, and D. J. Nutta. "Neural Correlates of the Psychedelic State as Determined by fMRI Studies with Psilocybin." *Proceedings of the National Academy of Sciences* 109 (2012): 2138–43.

LSD fMRI: Carhart-Harris, R. L., S. Muthukumaraswamy, L. Roseman, M. Kaelen, W. Droog, K. Murphy, E. Tagliazucchi, E. E. Schenberg, T. Nest, C. Orban, R. Leech, L. Williams, M. Bolstridge, B. Sessa, J. MacGonigle, M. I. Sereno, D. Nichols, P. J. Hellyer, P. Hobden, J. Evans, K. D. Singh, R. G. Wise, H. V. Curran, A. Feilding, and D. J. Nutta. "Neural Correlates of the LSD Experience Revealed by Multimodal Neuroimaging." *Proceedings of the National Academy of Sciences* 113 (2016): 4853–8.

MDMA: Meyer, J. S. "3,4-Methylenedioxymethamphetamine (MDMA): Current Perspectives." *Substance Abuse and Rehabilitation* 4 (2013): 83–99.

Ketamine and depression: Lener, M.S., M. J. Niciu, E. D. Ballard, M. Park, L. T. Park, A. C. Nugent, and C. A. Zarat. "Glutamate and Gamma-Aminobutyric Acid Systems in the Pathophysiology of Major Depression and Antidepressant Response to Ketamine." *Biological Psychiatry* (2016). http://dx.doi.org/10.1016/j.biopsych.2016.05.005.

LSD and depression: dos Santos, R. G., F. L. Osório, J. A. S. Crippa, J. Riba, A. W. Zuardi, and J. E. C. Hallak. "Antidepressive, Anxiolytic, and Antiaddictive Effects of Ayahuasca, Psilocybin and Lysergic Acid Diethylamide (LSD): A Systematic Review of Clinical Trials Published in the Last 25 Years." *Therapeutic Advances in Psychopharmacology* 6 (2016): 193–213.

Test Your Understanding

Multiple-Choice

1. Which of the following is not part of the mechanism of 5-HT_{2A} receptors?
   a. activation of phospholipase C (PLC)
   b. phosphorylation of calcium channels
   c. activation of K^+ channels
   d. inhibition of glutamate release

2. The depersonalization produced by psychedelics is caused by
   a. increased connectivity between the visual and other sensory regions of the cortex
   b. blockage of communication between the anterior and posterior nodes of the DMN
   c. hyperstimulation of the visual sensory regions in the occipital lobes
   d. inhibition of the filtering function of the thalamus

3. Of the three dissociative anesthetics, which has the shortest duration of action?
   a. PCP
   b. ketamine
   c. dextromethorphan
   d. *Salvia divinorum*

4. The main mechanism of action of dissociative anesthetics is
   a. blocking NMDA receptors
   b. blocking nicotinic receptors
   c. blocking AMPA receptors
   d. blocking muscarinic receptors

5. Blocking muscarinic receptors in the occipital cortex causes
   a. clouding of consciousness
   b. inhibition of thalamic filtering
   c. drowsiness
   d. spontaneous visual stimulation and hallucinations

6. Anti-muscarinics are not frequently abused because
   a. they are difficult to obtain
   b. they don't produce euphoria
   c. they produce side effects by blocking the parasympathetic nervous system
   d. all of the above

7. MDMA causes the release of oxytocin from the
   a. hypothalamus
   b. nucleus accumbens
   c. RAS
   d. VTA

8. Stimulant hallucinogens are called such because of their effect on
   a. norepinephrine and dopamine receptors
   b. dopamine and muscarinic receptors
   c. muscarinic and serotonin receptors
   d. serotonin and norepinephrine receptors

Essay Questions

1. Depersonalization is important to the spiritual aspects of psychedelics such as LSD and psilocybin. What is depersonalization, and why might it produce spiritual growth?
2. Why are dissociative anesthetics considered to be dirty drugs? How does this explain differences between them?
3. One hypothesis of how anti-muscarinic hallucinogens produce delirium is by inhibiting the thalamic-filtering process. How do they do this, and how does this action cause delirium?
4. What is a designer drug?
5. Compare and contrast MDMA and mescaline.

Credits

- Fig. 11.0: Copyright © by Depositphotos / Albisoima.
- Fig. 11.1a: Copyright © 2003 by burgkirsch / Wikimedia Commons, (CC BY-SA 2.5) at https://commons.wikimedia.org/wiki/File:Ergot01.jpg.
- Fig. 11.1b: Copyright © 2007 by Alan Rockefeller / Mushroom Observer, (CC BY-SA 3.0) at http://mushroomobserver.org/image/show_image/6514.
- Fig. 11.1c: Copyright © 2006 by Charles Bikle / Erowid. Reprinted with permission.
- Fig. 11.1d: Copyright © 2005 by Heah / Wikimedia Commons, (CC BY-SA 3.0) at https://commons.wikimedia.org/wiki/File:Aya-cooking.jpg.
- Fig. 11.3: Psychonaught / Wikimedia Commons / Copyright in the Public Domain.
- Fig. 11.5: Copyright © by Depositphotos / Albisoima.
- Fig. 11.7a: U.S. Drug Enforcement Agency / Copyright in the Public Domain.
- Fig. 11.7b: U.S. Department of Justice / Copyright in the Public Domain.
- Fig. 11.7c: Psychonaught / Wikimedia Commons / Copyright in the Public Domain.
- Fig. 11.8a: Copyright © 2009 by H. Zell / Wikimedia Commons, (CC BY-SA 3.0) at https://commons.wikimedia.org/wiki/File:Datura_stramonium_002.JPG.
- Fig. 11.8b: Copyright © 2010 by Donald Macauley, (CC BY-SA 2.0) at https://commons.wikimedia.org/wiki/File:Flickr_-_don_macauley_-_Deadly_Nightshade.jpg.
- Fig. 11.8c: Copyright © 2014 by Mikenorton / Wikimedia Commons, (CC BY-SA 3.0) at https://commons.wikimedia.org/wiki/File:Henbane2.jpg.
- Fig. 11.8d: Copyright © 2006 by tato grasso / Wikimedia Commons, (CC BY-SA 2.5) at https://commons.wikimedia.org/wiki/File:Mandragora_autumnalis1432.JPG.
- Fig. 11.10a: U.S. Drug Enforcement Agency / Copyright in the Public Domain.
- Fig. 11.10b: Copyright © 2011 by CostaPPPR / Wikimedia Commons, (CC BY-SA 3.0) at https://commons.wikimedia.org/wiki/File:Lophophora-williamsii-costapppr.jpg.

Solution Key

Chapter 1

Multiple-Choice

1. a, 2. c, 3. d, 4. d, 5. b, 6. d, 7. a, 8. d

Essay Questions

1. A drug injected intramuscularly (IM) is first absorbed into the capillaries. From there it goes into the venous circulation, and to the right side of the heart. The heart pumps it into the pulmonary circuit, where it passes through the lungs, and back to the left side of the heart. The heart then pumps it to the systemic circuit, some of which goes to the brain.

2. The kidneys remove toxins from the blood. They do this by filtering all dissolved chemicals out of the blood in Bowman's capsule and then reabsorbing salts and nutrients that are important to conserve. This locks polar toxins in the urine and results in them being excreted. The liver helps in the process by making nonpolar compounds more polar, allowing the kidneys to remove them.

3. Because these drugs are antidiarrheal medicines, they must work in the peripheral nervous system, that is, the autonomic nerves that stimulate or inhibit the large intestine. However, because they produce none of the central effects of morphine or heroin, they must not be activating the opiate receptors in the brain. Therefore, the reason these are safe opiates is that they most likely do not pass the blood-brain barrier and get into the brain.

4. Snorted drugs are very rapidly taken into the body and reach a high peak. Orally consumed drugs enter the body slowly and don't peak as high. This is because orally consumed drugs have a longer path to take before absorption (stomach, then small intestine), and much of the drug is metabolized via the liver (first-pass effect). The person who snorted is the one who overdoses.

5. There are two main reasons why a drug can be detected in the urine long after its effects have worn off. One is that many drugs are nonpolar and sequester into fatty tissues. This decreases their concentration in the blood and also produces a long detection half-life as the drugs slowly leach out of the fat and into the blood for removal by the kidneys. The second reason is that detection methods for drugs and drug metabolites in the urine are very sensitive; they are much more sensitive than the potency of the drugs.

Chapter 2

Multiple-Choice

1. b, 2. a, 3. c, 4. b, 5. c, 6. d, 7. b, 8. a

Essay Questions

1. In a neuron, Na^+ is very low inside and K^+ is very high inside. This asymmetric distribution of ions is used to set up a membrane potential and produce action potentials. The membrane potential is produced by allowing a small amount of K^+ to leave the cell through K^+ leak channels, leaving the inside of the cell slightly negative (about -70 mV).

The action potential is then produced when the cell is stimulated and VDNa⁺Cs open. This allows Na⁺ to enter the cell (down its concentration gradient), which depolarizes the membrane. Milliseconds later, VDNa⁺Cs inactivate and VDK⁺Cs then open, allowing K⁺ to leave, repolarizing the cell. Once the cell is repolarized, the VDK⁺Cs close again.

2. An excitatory postsynaptic potential (EPSP) is a depolarizing pulse, which makes the cell less negative. This is excitatory because it promotes an AP in the postsynaptic membrane. It is produced by Na⁺ entering the cell via ligand-gated channels. An inhibitory postsynaptic potential (IPSP) is a hyperpolarizing pulse, which makes the cell more negative. This inhibits an action potential in the postsynaptic membrane. It is produced by either K⁺ leaving or Cl⁻ entering through ligand-gated channels.

3. Action potentials are initiated by the opening of VDNa⁺Cs. When these are blocked, sensory neurons are unable to generate action potentials to relay sensory information to the brain.

4. Action potentials are all-or-nothing because of the threshold effect produced by the K⁺ leak channels. Depolarizing stimuli open VDNa⁺Cs, allowing in Na⁺ and producing more depolarization. If this Na⁺ entry is less than the K⁺ exit via the K⁺ leak channels, the membrane repolarizes—in other words, "nothing" happens. If, on the other hand, the depolarizing stimulus opens enough VDNa⁺Cs to supersede the K⁺ leak channels, it will open more VDNa⁺Cs, leading to more depolarization. This produces a positive feedback loop that opens all of the VDNa⁺Cs—in other words, "all" of it happens.

5. The soma determines the frequency of APs that are generated in the axon. It does this by adding together the incoming EPSPs and IPSPs from the dendrites and relaying this information to the axon hillock. The more EPSPs there are, the greater the frequency of action potentials in the axon. IPSPs subtract from the EPSPs and decrease the frequency of APs. If Valium increases the effect of the IPSPs by increasing Cl⁻ current, this will decrease the frequency of APs in the axon.

Chapter 3

Multiple-Choice

1. c, 2. d, 3. a, 4. a, 5. d, 6. b, 7. d, 8. c

Essay Questions

1. The terminal bulb of the axon stores neurotransmitters in vesicles near the membrane. When the action potential reaches here, it opens voltage-dependent Ca^{2+} channels. The influx of Ca^{2+} causes vesicles to fuse with the plasma membrane. Neurotransmitters are released into the synaptic cleft.

2. There are several possible mechanisms by which this could work. The toxin (omega conotoxin) actually blocks the voltage-dependent Ca^{2+} channels in the axon bulb. This blocks transmission because entry of Ca^{2+} into the axon bulb is the trigger for neurotransmitter release. The toxin could theoretically block the internal response to Ca^{2+}. It could do this by blocking the binding of Ca^{2+} to the proteins on the vesicle that respond to

it or by disrupting the proteins involved in fusing the vesicles to the plasma membrane (as botulinum toxin does). It could block the forward movement of vesicles. These are four general mechanisms that would apply to all axon bulbs.

3. A G-protein coupled receptor can affect the postsynaptic membrane in three different ways. The G-protein may directly open an ion channel. This skips all the downstream steps and provides very fast transmission. A G-protein may produce cAMP, and this may directly interact with a channel. This involves one more step; therefore, it is a little slower. Finally, the kinase that is activated by cAMP may phosphorylate an ion channel. This is the slowest of the three mechanisms because it involves the most number of steps; however, it lasts the longest and is involved in memory.

4. If a drug allowed Ca^{2+} to enter a synaptic bulb freely, the synaptic bulb would dump its entire contents of NT into the synapse at once. This is because Ca^{2+} is the trigger for the fusing of the NT-containing vesicles with the membrane. Ca^{2+} entry is controlled by the voltage-dependent Ca^{2+} channel, which is opened and closed by action potentials. If Ca^{2+} entry is not controlled, all vesicles will fuse and dump.

5. When a person first smokes cigarettes, he or she has a normal number of nicotinic receptors in his or her body. The added nicotine overstimulates these receptors, producing an extreme effect. Once cigarette smoking becomes a habit, the body responds to the chronic overstimulation by decreasing the number of nicotinic receptors available. This moderates the effects of the nicotine so that the response is not as extreme. However, when a chronic smoker stops taking in nicotine, the body now does not have enough receptors to respond to the normal amount of endogenous neurotransmitter (acetylcholine) to maintain a normal homeostasis. The result is withdrawal symptoms that cause the person to smoke again to obtain relief.

Chapter 4

Multiple-Choice

1. d, 2. b, 3. c, 4. a, 5. a, 6. b, 7. d, 8. c

Essay Questions

1. The cerebellum is involved in error-checking during movement. It has stored memories of how a body should be positioned at rest (postural) and in motion. It receives sensory information about the body's position and checks this against its memories of where it should be and makes subtle corrections to maintain balance and smoothen movements. Without a cerebellum, a person would have jerky, uncoordinated movement and would be unable to maintain a steady posture.

2. The thalamus is centrally located and coordinates the ascending and descending tracts in the brain. It receives motor instructions from the cortex and relays these to the basal ganglia and pons to control movement. It also receives sensory information and sends it to the proper region of the cortex to be processed. Another important role is to filter the incoming sensory information to focus attention on the most important stimuli while ignoring stimuli of less importance.

3. The medulla in the brain stem is responsible for autonomic functions: respiration, blood pressure, heart rate, digestion, coughing, and vomiting. These are all vital to survival on a minute-to-minute basis. Drugs that affect these areas (opiates, alcohol, etc.) depress these functions and can cause death. The cerebral cortex is involved with sensory perceptions and cognition. While important, these functions are not vital to short-term survival (as long as you don't jump off a building).

4. The reticular activating system (RAS) is a bundle of neurons in the hindbrain that relays stimulus to the cortex and the rest of the brain. The RAS regulates arousal (sleep vs. wake cycles) as well as alertness, attention, and excitement. The primary neurotransmitters used by the RAS are acetylcholine and norepinephrine, which increase wakefulness. For this reason, the drug in question probably is an antagonist of one or the other of these receptors.

5. Hallucinogens affect the cerebral cortex, which is the outermost layer of the cerebrum. The cerebral cortex receives and processes sensory input, interprets information, and decides on voluntary movement. It is the center for vision, hearing, speech, sensory perception, and emotion. Part of this is called the prefrontal cortex. This part doesn't directly receive sensory input or directly create movement, but stores memories, controls complex behaviors, processes information, and makes decisions. This is the thinking part of the brain, where rationality is controlled. Drugs that affect these areas interact with acetylcholine, anandamide (cannabinoid), and serotonin receptors, as well as glutamate receptors, which are in all areas of the brain.

Chapter 5

Multiple-Choice

1. b, 2. a, 3. d, 4. d, 5. d, 6. a, 7. d, 8. d

Essay Questions

1. The Skinner box was important because it showed how behavior could be modified by reward or punishment. This experiment could condition a rat to perform a specific behavior in return for a treat, which we now know produced pleasure in the brain. The experiment of Olds and Milner replaced the external treat with direct stimulation of the brain. By moving the electrode around, they were able to directly map the structures that are responsible for euphoria and therefore addiction.

2. The limbic system, which includes the amygdala, hippocampus, dorsal striatum (DS), nucleus accumbens (NA), and cerebral cortex, is the major reward center of the brain. The amygdala is the center of emotions. The NA produces the feeling of euphoria or reward that is usually sought by drug takers. The hippocampus is the site of short-term storage of memories. These memories are later erased or moved to long-term storage in the cerebral cortex. The DS is the site of habit formation. The combination of reward, habit, emotion, and memory makes this system the center of the addiction potential of drugs; rewarding experiences are remembered and repeated.

3. Dopamine is especially important for two things in the brain: movement and reward. An antagonist of dopamine receptors would probably produce effects similar to Parkinson's disease, that is, the inability to

initiate movement. It would probably also block any pleasure, which is a condition called anhedonia.

4. Someone with RDS would have a difficult time experiencing pleasure from normal, everyday life. The stimulation produced by drugs may be the only way that the person can feel pleasure. This would make drugs a stronger motivator for this person than it would for the average person who can experience joy normally.

5. The emotional set point of mood is created by a balance between reward and anti-reward pathways. It provides a baseline from which external stimuli can make a person feel better or worse, thus motivating behavior. Addicts become neuroadapted to the presence of the supranormal stimulation of the drug by decreasing the baseline activity of the reward pathway and increasing the baseline activity of the anti-reward pathway. This results in a lower baseline emotional set point in the absence of the drug; the person feels depressed and anxious in its absence and needs the drug to come back up to normal functioning. This is called dependence.

Chapter 6

Multiple-Choice

1. d, 2. b, 3. d, 4. a, 5. c, 6. a, 7. c, 8. b

Essay Questions

1. EEG recordings are very inexpensive and easy to make. They also have excellent time resolution, in the order of milliseconds. Unfortunately, the geographical isolation of the method is weak; it measures electrical activity over broad areas, and pinpointing active areas is not possible. In addition, it can measure only from the surface of the cortex and a short distance into the fissures. These drawbacks limit its utility.

2. The SN is the central hub of cognition. It receives external cues and information about internal states and error checks these. In this way, it decides whether cognition should be dominated by TPN or DNM and switched over to the appropriate network.

3. The cortex detects time passing through a coordination between the DMN and the movement centers lower in the brain (basal ganglia and cerebellum). When a person is focused on a task, he or she is using the TPN. When the TPN is activated, the DMN is suppressed by anti-correlation. Because the DMN is that part that senses time, a person on task loses this sense.

4. The anterior part of the DMN (the MPC) is the executive-function portion. This does the actual thinking of the DMN. The posterior portions (the LPL, precuneus, and PCC) store self-referential memories and memories of places, and relay this information to the MPC. This process produces the sense of self, as distinct from the environment, in a place and a time. If the connection is lost, the thinking will go on but will be separate from memories of the self. This causes an out-of-body feeling and a loss of the sense of time (which is also a function of the DMN).

5. During normal development, there is a segregation of the SN and DMN; connection between the anterior part of the cingulate cortex (ACC) and its posterior part (PC) is decreased. At the same time,

the connections within the networks are strengthened. In ADHD, this doesn't occur to the same extent. The result is that the person with ADHD has a hard time staying in TPN; self-referential thinking and mind wandering (DMN) continually intrude and tax attentional resources.

Chapter 7

Multiple-Choice

1. d, 2. a, 3. d, 4. a, 5. a, 6. d, 7. b, 8. b

Essay Questions

1. The BAC for a given amount of alcohol is affected by stomach contents and the rate of drinking. Stomach contents slow down absorption, which occurs mainly in the small intestine. Keeping the alcohol in the stomach allows more time for the ADH there to break it down. Also, the faster a person drinks, the higher his or her BAC will be for the same amount of alcohol. This is because the liver has a chance to break down circulating alcohol if a person drinks slowly, as opposed to rapid drinking, where the alcohol is all absorbed at once; this effect also decreases BAC when drinking on a full stomach. BAC is affected by a person's size and body fat percentage. Both of these factors affect the volume of distribution of the alcohol. Body fat percentage decreases the volume of distribution because alcohol is excluded from fatty tissues. Carbonation can increase BAC, as the gas released in the stomach increases pressure, which increases

gastric emptying. Previous exposure to alcohol decreases BAC, as ADH is upregulated by exposure to alcohol, increasing its metabolism. Finally, BAC is affected by sex. Women will have a higher BAC than men will for the same amount of alcohol consumed for several reasons.

2. Low-dose alcohol does three specific things. It potentiates the activation of GABA receptors by GABA. This increases IPSPs all over the brain. It also affects glutamate by blocking glutamate receptors and inhibiting glutamate release. These mechanisms decrease EPSPs all over the brain. High-dose alcohol produces a nonspecific effect. It dissolves into phospholipid membranes and disturbs the function of proteins there, including ion channels. This has the effect of shutting down neurons.

3. Alcohol is an anxiolytic that inhibits cognitive function. One of the effects of this is a decrease in inhibitions. Alcohol decreases a person's awareness of his or her environment and social situation, and reduces the anxiety about the consequences of behavior. Because of this, alcohol can make people feel more relaxed in social situations, allowing them to exhibit behavior that they would otherwise be too anxious to display.

4. In all likelihood, an older, heavier man would be able to consume more alcohol than a younger, thinner woman would. The man would probably have a larger volume of distribution, both because of his larger size and his sex. Also, being older, he would probably have a higher tolerance for alcohol. However, this could be the woman's advantage. She may be a chronic alcoholic with a very high tolerance for alcohol. This would allow her to win the contest and still be sober enough to clean up the bar.

5. Cirrhosis of the liver is a degenerative liver disease caused by chronic, high-dose alcohol consumption. It begins with a fatty liver, in which liver cells store large vacuoles of fat. This causes stress on the cells and inflammation. If alcohol abuse continues, the inflammation causes cells to die and be replaced by scar tissue. This condition proceeds to alcoholic hepatitis. In the long term, the process continues until a majority of liver cells have been replaced by scar tissue. This is cirrhosis of the liver.

Chapter 8

Multiple-Choice

1. c, 2. c, 3. a, 4. d, 5. d, 6. b, 7. c, 8. a

Essay Questions

1. Morphine is the opioid isolated from the natural source, the opium poppy. It is mostly polar in the pH of the bloodstream, which makes it slowly enter the brain to produce its effects. Heroin is morphine that is chemically modified to make it less polar by adding two acyl groups. This allows it easy entry into the brain. However, heroin is not active on MORs. Instead, heroin is metabolized into morphine in the brain.

2. Methadone is a MOR agonist with a slow onset of effect and a very long half-life. It is used as a maintenance drug for addicts because the slow onset eliminates the rush seen in nonpolar opioids (heroin), which is addictive and makes everyday life difficult. Also, the long half-life decreases the peaks and troughs produced by repeated injection of fast-acting opioids, decreasing withdrawal symptoms. It is not a cure; it is meant to moderate the debilitating effect of opioids and help the addict conduct more normal life.

3. Disinhibition is the blocking of an inhibitory input. GABA-releasing neurons in the NA inhibit the release of dopamine, which is feedback to decrease euphoria. Endorphin-releasing axons from the hypothalamus activate MORs on the GABAergic axon bulbs (axoaxonic synapses). MOR activation inhibits the production of cAMP in the axon bulb, which decreases PAK phosphorylation of the VDCC. This decreases GABA release, indirectly increasing dopamine release. Thus, endorphins block the inhibitory effect of GABA, disinhibiting the release of dopamine.

4. There are two drugs that instantly block the effects of heroin: Narcan (naloxone) and Nalline (nalorphine). They are antagonists of opioid receptors. They bind to MORs and block their effect. By doing this, they can instantly stop the effects of the opioid and bring an overdosing individual back to life.

5. Overstimulated opioid receptors are rapidly downregulated. This diminishes the effect of the drugs. As a result, users increase their dose to try to achieve the euphoria that they experienced before the receptors became downregulated by increasing the dose. Because heroin on the street is not regulated, the dose is not controlled, and the drug may even be cut with other drugs (e.g., fentanyl) to increase its effect. This, combined with the narrow window of effect/toxicity for heroin means that users often misjudge the dose needed and overdose.

Chapter 9

Multiple-Choice

1. b, 2. c, 3. b, 4. d, 5. b, 6. a, 7. a, 8. d

Essay Questions

1. Cocaine HCl (powder cocaine) is the water-soluble form of cocaine. It is charged and therefore poorly absorbed. It is usually snorted, but sometimes injected. Powdered cocaine decomposes with heat and can't be smoked. Freebase cocaine (crack) is crystallized. The hydrochloride form is treated with base and extracted into organic solvent to form crack. Because it is nonpolar, it is easily absorbed. It is heat stable and is usually smoked.

2. These drugs both produce intense euphoria by increasing dopamine in the nucleus accumbens (NA). This is seen by the prefrontal cortex (PFC) as a supranormal stimulus. This means that is has extremely high salience, preferable to any other stimuli. Neuroadaptation causes an increased connection between the PFC and the NA, creating craving, and between the dorsal striatum and the NA, producing compulsive behavior.

3. TAAR1 is a G-protein coupled receptor found on the plasma membrane of some axon bulbs. It activates G_s to stimulate adenylyl cyclase, increasing cAMP in the axon bulb. Elevation of cAMP activates protein kinase A (PKA), which phosphorylates voltage-dependent calcium channels (VDCCs), increasing the influx of calcium during action potentials; this increases vesicle fusion and neurotransmitter release. PKA also phosphorylates the amine pump, causing its internalization, and inhibiting its function. In addition, by activating protein kinase C, the amine pump is phosphorylated on a different site, reversing its function. This is true of the amine pump on neurotransmitter storage vesicles as well. This causes the neurotransmitters to be pumped out of the vesicles into the cytoplasm and then out of the cytoplasm into the synapse. The result is a massive release of dopamine, norepinephrine, and serotonin.

4. A common problem in ADHD is the inability to inactivate the DMN when attempting to focus on a task. This lack of anti-correlation between the DMN and TPN causes distracting thoughts to intrude. The amphetamines increase dopamine release, which causes a decreased connectivity between the SN and the DMN, making it easier to shift into TPN and suppress self-referential thoughts.

5. There are two main reasons that the euphoria of cocaine diminishes. One is that cocaine doesn't directly stimulate dopamine receptors, but inhibits the reuptake of dopamine. Eventually the axon terminals become depleted of dopamine, and euphoria is no longer felt; the user keeps using to maintain the stimulant effect, which is produced by norepinephrine. Also, continual overstimulation of the dopamine receptors by inhibiting dopamine reuptake causes downregulation of the receptors, diminishing the effect of any dopamine that is released.

Chapter 10

Multiple-Choice

1. a, 2. d, 3. d, 4. b and d, 5. b, 6. a, 7. b, 8. c

Essay Questions

1. Inhalation, whether by smoking or vaporizing the source, is a much faster means of absorption than oral ingestion. Inhaled THC peaks in ten minutes, whereas ingested edibles may take as long as two to three hours to peak. Inhalation is a more efficient mechanism of absorption, with up to 50% of the inhaled THC being absorbed. Oral ingestion confronts both stomach digestion and first-pass metabolism; bioavailability is between 4 and 12%. However, 10% of the absorbed THC is converted into 11-OH-THC, which is psychoactive and more potent than THC. Because of the differences in absorption, inhaled THC peaks much faster and higher than when it is orally consumed. However, orally consumed THC will produce a longer-lasting effect.

2. 2-AG is synthesized by the action of phospholipase C (PLC) and diacylglycerol lipase (DAGL). PLC cleaves off the polar head group of a membrane phospholipid, releasing diacylglycerol (DAG). One of the two fatty acids groups of DAG is cleaved off by DAGL, producing 2-AG. 2-AG diffuses out of the presynaptic cell and across the synapse, and interacts with CB1 receptors on the presynaptic membrane. 2-AG will eventually be transported back into the presynaptic cell by an uptake pump and metabolized into arachidonic acid and glycerol by monoacylglycerol lipase (MAGL).

3. CB1 receptors are found on presynaptic membranes in synapses. When an agonist is bound to them they activate the G protein G_i, which inhibits the production of cAMP in the presynaptic axon bulb. The decrease in cAMP concentration inhibits protein kinase A, which normally stimulates the voltage-dependent calcium channel (VDCC) through phosphorylation. As a result of less phosphorylation of the channel, less Ca^{2+} enters during an action potential. CB1 receptors also directly inhibit VDCCs through G_q. Finally, CB1 receptors also activate K^+ channels; this limits the depolarization during action potentials, decreasing Ca^{2+} entry through the VDCC. As a result of these three mechanisms, less neurotransmitter is released from the presynaptic axon bulb. The main neurotransmitter affected is glutamate, although acetylcholine (in nicotinic synapses) and GABA are also affected.

4. THC is anxiolytic, decreasing stress and anxiety and increasing positive emotions by activation of CB1 receptors in the amygdala. Activation of CB1 receptors may be involved in the extinction of conditioned fear, that is, losing a fearful feeling that builds up in response to repetitive negative stimuli. This is the type of stimulus that causes PTSD. THC has the potential to inhibit this unnatural buildup of fear.

5. fMRI brain scans of chronic users show decreases in gray matter in the orbitofrontal cortex, which is in the MPC and part of the DMN. DTI brain scans show increased white matter (axon tracts) connecting the MPC to the limbic system, suggesting hyperactivity in this pathway. Chronic cannabis users are characterized as being indecisive, as having a short attention span and brief working memory, and as leading a lethargic, sedentary lifestyle. The decrease in gray matter in this important executive decision–making area correlates with the indecision and memory deficiency. Increased MPC-limbic functional connectivity suggests inability to focus on a task (short attention span) and increased emotional-DMN processing, which is similar to that seen in depression.

Thus, amotivational syndrome (lethargy, lack of goal-directed activity) may be associated with this increased MPC-limbic connectivity.

Chapter 11

Multiple-Choice

1. c, 2. b, 3. b, 4. a, 5. b, 6. c, 7. a, 8. d

Essay Questions

1. Depersonalization refers to the loss of the sense of self. Sense of self is primarily a DMN construct. The executive regions in the anterior nodes of the DMN (medial prefrontal cortex, MPC) communicate with posterior regions (precuneus and lateral parietal lobe) to retrieve long-term, self-referential memories, spatial memories (putting the person in a time and place), and autobiographical memories. The MPC puts these memories into the current context to provide awareness. Psychedelics separate the anterior and posterior nodes of the DMN, so the MPC can no longer access who the person is or separate the person from his or her environment. Thus, the person no longer senses himself or herself as separate from the environment but as one with the environment. This is what creates the sense of spiritual growth. It halts the self-referential thinking and causes the person to see himself or herself as a small part of the wider world.

2. Dissociative anesthetics are considered dirty because they affect many receptors. Their main mechanism of action is to block NMDA receptors, but they can also affect dopamine, acetylcholine, serotonin, and opioid neurotransmission, as well as voltage-dependent sodium and calcium channels. Each drug has different secondary receptors that it affects and a different potency for each of these receptors. This is why the main mechanism is the same for all three examples, yet they can have different effects.

3. This hypothesis concerns how the filtering process of the thalamus is modulated by the limbic system. The filtering makes sure that only important sensory information makes it to the prefrontal cortex (PFC). Filtering is increased (i.e., sensory information is blocked) by neurons from the striatum that release GABA in the thalamus. Other neurons in the striatum release acetylcholine onto muscarinic receptors on the GABAergic neurons to stimulate them to increase filtering by the thalamus. The acetylcholine neurons are, in turn, stimulated by the PFC to provide feedback to the amount of sensory information it receives, keeping it within the range of what the PFC can handle. Thus, muscarinic receptors are a link in the chain to increase filtering in the thalamus to protect the PFC's cognitive resources. Antimuscarinic drugs block the stimulation of the GABAergic neurons. The result is less filtering of sensory information, and consciousness is overwhelmed. The result is cognitive confusion (delirium) and hallucinations.

4. Designer drugs are compounds synthesized to stay ahead of legal restrictions on drugs of abuse. Chemists making these drugs typically start with the structure of norepinephrine and change it in some novel way by adding different functional groups to the structure. This produces a new compound that is not currently illegal to make and sell. The drugs that are made usually have novel effects as

well, combining the effects of the monoamine neurotransmitters (norepinephrine, dopamine, and serotonin) in different ways.

5. MDMA and mescaline are both taken orally and have a long latency to effect (more than one hour). Mescaline lasts longer, producing effects for up to ten hours, whereas MDMA lasts three to four hours. This is because MDMA is more readily metabolized by the liver. Both drugs have stimulatory, hallucinogenic, and euphoric effects. They do this by affecting norepinephrine, serotonin, and (to a lesser extent) dopamine receptors. However, their mechanisms of action are different. MDMA blocks reuptake of neurotransmitters and reverses their presynaptic amine pumps. This dumps neurotransmitters out of presynaptic vesicles and then out of the axon bulbs, flooding the synapse. Mescaline is an agonist of these receptors, directly producing its result. Another difference is the drugs' effect on serotonin. Because MDMA dumps serotonin out of axon bulbs, it has effects on both $5\text{-}HT_{1A}$ and $5\text{-}HT_{2A}$ receptors. $5\text{-}HT_{1A}$ receptors release oxytocin from the hypothalamus, increasing empathy and social bonding. Mescaline affects mainly $5\text{-}HT_{2a}$ receptors, producing more vivid visual hallucinations than MDMA does.

Abbreviations/ Acronyms

- 2-AG: 2-arachidonoyl glycerol
- 5-HT: 5-hydroxytryptamine
- 7-TMRs: seven-transmembrane receptors
- 11-OH-THC: 11-hydroxy-Δ9-tetrahydrocannabinol
- AC: adenylyl cyclase
- ACC: anterior cingulate cortex
- ACTH: adrenocorticotropic hormone
- ADH: alcohol dehydrogenase
- ADH: antidiuretic hormone
- ADHD: attention deficient hyperactivity disorder
- AEA: anandamide
- ALDH: aldehyde dehydrogenase
- AMPA: α-amino-3-hydroxy-5-methyl-4-isoxazolepropionic acid
- AP: action potential
- ARND: alcohol-related neurodevelopmental disorder
- ASD: autism spectrum disorder
- BAC: blood alcohol content
- BBB: blood-brain barrier
- BOLD: blood-oxygen-level dependent
- cAMP: cyclic adenosine monophosphate
- carboxy-THC: 11-nor-9-carboxy-delta-9-tetrahydrocannabinol
- CB1: cannabinoid receptor 1
- CB2: cannabinoid receptor 2
- CBD: cannabidiol
- CNS: central nervous system
- CRF: corticotropin-releasing factor
- CTZ: chemical trigger zone
- DAG: diacylglycerol
- DAGL: diacylglycerol lipase
- DLPC: dorsolateral prefrontal cortex
- DMN: default-mode network
- DMT: dimethyltryptamine
- DORs: delta opioid receptors
- DRG: dorsal root ganglia
- DS: dorsal striatum
- *DSM*: *Diagnostic and Statistical Manual of Mental Disorders*
- DTI: diffusion tensor imaging
- DXM: dextromethorphan
- EEG: electroencephalography
- EPSP: excitatory postsynaptic potential
- FAAH: fatty acid amide hydrolase
- GABA: gamma-aminobutyric acid
- GPCRs: G-protein coupled receptors
- FAS: fetal alcohol syndrome
- fMRI: functional magnetic resonance imaging
- HCl: hydrochloric acid
- HPA: hypothalamus-pituitary-adrenal
- HPPD: hallucinogen persisting perception disorder
- IM: intramuscular
- IPSP: inhibitory postsynaptic potential
- IV: intravenous
- KORs: kappa opioid receptors
- LPL: lateral parietal lobe
- LSD: lysergic acid diethylamide
- MAGL: monoacylglycerol lipase
- MAO-A: monoamine oxidase A
- MDMA: 3,4-methylenedioxymethamphetamine
- MEG: magnetoencephalography
- MORs: mu opioid receptors
- MPC: medial prefrontal cortex
- NA: nucleus accumbens
- NMDA: N-methyl-D-aspartate
- NSAIDs: nonsteroidal anti-inflammatory drugs
- NT: neurotransmitter
- PAG: periaqueductal gray matter
- PAHs: polyaromatic hydrocarbons
- PCC: posterior cingulate cortex
- PCP: phencyclidine
- PDE: phosphodiesterase

- PET: positron emission tomography
- pFAS: partial fetal alcohol syndrome
- PFC: prefrontal cortex
- PKA: protein kinase A
- PKC: protein kinase C
- PLC: phospholipase C
- PNS: peripheral nervous system
- PPC: posterior parietal cortex
- PTSD: posttraumatic stress disorder
- RAS: reticular activating system
- RDS: reward deficiency syndrome
- SC: subcutaneous
- SN: salience network
- SSRIs: selective serotonin reuptake inhibitors
- TAAR1: trace amine-associated receptor 1
- THC: Δ9-tetrahydrocannabinol
- THCA: tetrahydrocannabinolic acid
- THC-COOH: 11-nor-9-carboxy-delta-9-tetrahydrocannabinol
- TI: therapeutic index
- TPN: task-positive network
- VDCCs: voltage-dependent calcium channels
- VTA: ventral tegmental area

CPSIA information can be obtained
at www.ICGtesting.com
Printed in the USA
LVHW061134130822
725835LV00003B/34

9 781516 504411